AWAKEN NOW

TRANSFORM YOUR BODY, BRAIN, AND BRILLIANCE
WITH THE POWER OF HEALTH BY DESIGN

DR. MARINA DABCEVIC
LAC, DAOM, IFMCP

AWAKEN NOW

Transform Your Body, Brain, and Brilliance with the Power of Health by Design

Copyright © 2025. Marina Dabcevic. All rights reserved. No part of this publication may be reproduced, distributed, or transmitted in any form or by any means, including photocopying, recording, or other electronic or mechanical methods, without the prior written permission of the publisher, except in the case of brief quotations embodied in critical reviews and certain other noncommercial uses permitted by copyright law.

Awaken Now
1410 2nd Street, Ste 302
Santa Monica, CA, 90401
www.awakennowhealth.com

ISBN: 979-8-9931662-5-4

Book Design by Transcendent Publishing
Editing by Mary Rembert
Author Photography by Steven McNiel

Disclaimer: Although every effort has been made to ensure the accuracy and completeness of the information in this book, the author does not assume responsibility or liability for any errors, omissions, or outcomes that may result from its use. All content is provided for informational purposes only and is not a substitute for professional advice: medical, legal, financial, fitness, or otherwise. Readers are encouraged to seek guidance from qualified professionals regarding any questions or concerns. Health and fitness information contained herein is not intended to diagnose, treat, cure, or prevent any condition or disease. Always consult a licensed physician or healthcare provider before beginning any exercise program or addressing health-related concerns, and participate at your own risk.

Furthermore, the author makes no guarantees regarding the success or results readers may achieve by following any advice, strategies, or examples presented. Individual outcomes will vary based on personal circumstances, effort, and other factors, and any testimonials or examples represent exceptional results rather than typical experiences. By using this book, you voluntarily assume all risks and agree to release and discharge the author and publisher from any and all claims, known or unknown, arising from your reliance on the content. Your use of this book implies your acceptance of this disclaimer.

*"To attain excellence,
you must care more than others think is wise,
risk more than others think is safe,
dream more than others think is practical."*

–Unknown

Contents

Introduction 1

The Seven Core Biological Systems of Functional Medicine 5
    Core System 1: Assimilation. 6
    Core System 2: Defense and Repair. 10
    Core System 3: Energy 12
    Core System 4: Biotransformation and Elimination. 16
    Core System 5: Communication 20
    Core System 6: Transport 30
    Core System 7: Structural Integrity 33

Age Is Just a Number—But Which One? 47
    Biological Age vs. Chronological Age. 47
    Common Aging vs. Optimal Aging 50
    Why Do We Age? 51

The Blue Zones 53
    Let's Talk Diet. 54
    Let's Talk Movement. 56
    Let's Talk Family & Community 57
    Let's Talk Purpose. 59
    Let's Talk About Stress. 61

Rewire, Recharge, Reimagine 63
   Train the Mind, Heal the Body, Shift the Biology 63
   The Free Medicine You've Been Ignoring 66
   The Science of Seeing It Before You Become It 71

The Mirror Lies, Your Cells Don't. 73
   Biological Age Self Assessment (BASA) 73
   Medical Screening Symptoms Questionnaire 82

Beyond DNA: How Lifestyle Writes Your Genetic Story 89
   The Tale of Two Mice............................ 89
   Genetics vs. Epigenetics: The Game-Changer........... 90
   Enter: SNPs (Single Nucleotide Polymorphisms) 92
   Wait, What's Methylation, You Ask? 93
   So, What Can Mess With Methylation? 93
   Methylation: The Aging Accelerator or Slower-Downer?... 94
   Powering It All Are the Mitochondria (The Unsung Heroes).. 95
   Your Genes Are Listening 96
   Is One of Your Genes Acting Up? 106

Inflamed, Exhausted, or Anxious? Let's Talk Stress 127
   Good Stress (Eustress)............................ 127
   Bad Stress (Distress) 128

Eat Like You Love Yourself; Move Like You Mean It.......... 137
   What Your Plate Should Look Like:.................. 137
   Protein First..................................... 138
   Macronutrient Strategy........................... 139
   The Migrating Motor Complex (MMC) 139

Let's Talk Fasting................................. 140
Here's Your Ideal Eating Order:..................... 143
A Few Tips to Help You Break Free from Sugar 145
Eat the Rainbow, Literally! (Skittles NOT Included)..... 148

The Monthly Map: Eat, Move, and Thrive With Your Hormones.. 157
    For the Ladies (and Actually Men too, You All Have
        at Least One Female in Your Life—Pay Attention!) ... 157
    Why Cycle Syncing Matters After 40................ 158
    Four Phases 159

Hormone Disruptors: The Hidden Saboteurs in Your Daily Life... 165
    What Are Endocrine Disruptors?.................... 165
    Helpful Apps to Detox Your Life 171

Your Only Limit Is You 179
    Muscle Is the Organ of Longevity 179
    Functional Health Tests........................... 183

The Sleep Prescription.............................. 187
    Let's Talk About Sleep............................ 187

Pills with Purpose 195
    Let's Talk About Supplements 195

Spirit & Science: The Missing Link in Health 199
    Let's Talk Spirituality and Mindset................. 199
    Why Mindset Matters ... Scientifically 200
    A Little Brain Science............................ 200
    Train Your Mind Like an Athlete Trains Their Body 202
    "Nerve Cells That Fire Together, Wire Together" 202

Let's Talk Vibrations & Frequencies 205
The 5 Whys 211

And Here We Are ... The End (Or the Beginning) 215
Your Journey Doesn't End Here, It's Just Getting Started. . 217
Let's Keep Going Together 218
You're Not Meant to Do This Alone 219

Acknowledgments 223

About the Author 227

References 229

Dedication

To my entire family, my foundation, my joy, my safe place.

And especially to my kids, Parker and Bodie. You are in my heart and on my mind with every choice I make. Every step, every late night of work, every moment of learning and growing, all so I can be here with you, for as long as possible, to watch you grow, to cheer you on, and to love you through it all.

Introduction

Welcome to the rest of your life!

As a Board-certified Functional Medicine practitioner, licensed acupuncturist, and herbalist, I've spent the last 25 years working with patients in integrative health, and the last 14 immersed in the world of alternative and functional medicine.

What started as a personal healing journey has turned into a passionate mission through my California-based practice, Awaken Now Health, to help others worldwide reconnect with their bodies, rewire their minds, and reclaim their health.

Like many people, I didn't set out to be a healer. I was the kid who moved across the world, struggled with undiagnosed symptoms, and heard "it's all in your head" more times than I can count.

That frustration, and eventual awakening, led me to study everything from homeopathy to acupuncture, reflexology to functional medicine, and even frequency-specific microcurrent and peptide therapy.

This book is the culmination of all I've learned: the science, the spirit, and the systems that help us feel whole again. It's not about chasing perfection. It's about tuning into your body's needs, creating small shifts that add up to big change, and honoring your healing—physically, emotionally, mentally, and spiritually.

The road that brought me here wasn't easy. I didn't speak English when my family moved us from Croatia to Australia. I was teased because I had a thick accent, which I worked hard to get rid of. (Then I had to move to America so that I could have an accent again!)

I had glasses, braces, zero popularity, and the stress wrecked my digestion and breathing. I spent years going from doctor to doctor, having test after test, desperately trying to figure out what was wrong, only to be told, again and again, that it was all in my head.

And in a way it was. It was the stress, and it had a profound effect on my body, something no doctor could explain, but something I lived with every day. It wasn't until after high school that I began studying what actually fascinated me, meeting teachers and mentors who lit a fire in me and helped me realize how deeply the mind and body are connected.

I'll be honest, I barely made it through high school. I was working by 13, underpaid and overstretched, and my parents were rightfully worried I wouldn't amount to much.

But when I started learning on my own terms, when I found my purpose and passion, everything changed. I earned degrees, a doctorate, a couple of board certifications, and I kept learning, exploring every modality I could get my hands on, weaving together protocols that truly helped people heal.

That's what led me to write this book. I wanted to create something that addressed the full picture, not just diet, not just training, not just longevity, but the whole human experience: the body, mind, spirit, and everything in between.

Over the years, I've watched so many people struggle with their health, their hormones, their energy, and their mindset, all while trying to do "the right things" and still not feeling better.

I've learned that most people aren't lacking motivation; they're just missing a clear, compassionate roadmap. That's why I created a book and a membership program that feel clear, doable, and truly helpful. A place to turn when you feel off track, overwhelmed, or out of sync with yourself.

Inside this book, you'll find bite-sized insights that can create lasting change. You'll gain a deeper understanding of your physical body and, just as importantly, how your mind and spirit shape your health. You'll be introduced to both new ideas and familiar concepts, but with the dots finally connected.

You'll learn how to support your core systems: digestion, detox, stress response, hormones, mitochondria, and immune function, through simple, science-backed strategies.

You'll gain access to self-assessments, symptom maps, protocols, and lifestyle tools that empower you to make confident, informed decisions about your health. No fluff. Just real, lasting transformation.

Because here's the truth: your health is your greatest asset, and your time is just as valuable. If you don't invest in your wellness now, you may be forced to invest far more time, energy, and money into managing your disease later.

While that might sound intimidating to some of you, this book isn't about fear; it's about freedom, it's about understanding what's happening in your body, why it's happening, and what you can do about it.

Whether you're dealing with fatigue, brain fog, hormone imbalances, gut issues, or simply feeling off, this book is here to help you understand the "why" and take back control.

Use it as a guide, a workbook, and a mirror. Read it straight through or start with the chapters that speak to you most. Take the assessments, try the tools, and come back to it often. It's designed to evolve with you, to grow with your journey toward more clarity, energy, and alignment.

If you've been searching for answers, feeling stuck, or are just ready for something to change, this book is for you. You don't have to overhaul your entire life overnight. You just need to start where you are, listen to your body's wisdom, and take the next right step.

That's what this book is here to help you do.

So take a deep breath. You're exactly where you need to be.

Now, let's begin!

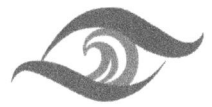

The Seven Core Biological Systems of Functional Medicine

First things first, let me introduce you to the seven core biological systems of Functional Medicine (go ahead, try saying that three times fast!). One of the biggest pitfalls of the Western medical system is the way it sends you straight to a specialist.

Now, don't get me wrong, specialists are amazing. But the problem? They usually see your condition only through the lens of their specialty. If they can't figure it out, they either hand you a medication (which, let's be honest, is often like playing target practice; sometimes you hit the bull's-eye, other times you're just throwing darts in the dark) or they refer you to another specialist.

Then that one does the exact same thing. Before you know it, you've got a lineup of specialists, each treating a symptom, and no one's talking to each other. No one's stepping back to look at you as a whole human being. OMG, okay, rant over.

In Functional Medicine, things work differently. Health and disease are viewed through the lens of a deeply interconnected and beautifully layered web of systems, not just isolated symptoms or individual organs.

The seven core biological systems are the foundation of this approach. These systems represent the major networks in the body that must work together in harmony to maintain health.

Functional Medicine practitioners use this systems-based model to:

- Find root causes of disease rather than treating just the symptoms
- Personalize treatment based on how systems interact
- Promote balance and optimal function across the body
- Have stronger connections with our patients
- Separate us from the standard medical doctor

When I can clearly see this beautiful web on a page in front of me, I can identify the dysfunctions in one or more of these systems, and that allows me to target lifestyle, nutrition, and medical interventions individually to restore optimum health.

Here are the seven core systems and why they are important. At the end of each section, you will get to do your first set of questionnaires that will give you an idea of whether you are healthy, severely imbalanced, or anything in between. Good luck!

Core System 1: Assimilation

Includes: Digestion, absorption, microbiome, and respiratory system

Why It's Important:

Assimilation is all about how the body takes in nutrients and oxygen, breaks them down, and absorbs them so they can actually be used. Sounds simple, right? I mean, we're breathing and eating all day, every day, and we don't even have to think about it.

But hold up ... how many of you hold your breath without realizing it? Or breathe only into your chest instead of your belly? And let's be honest, how many of us spend hours sitting at a computer, snacking on things that probably aren't doing us any favors?

When this system isn't functioning properly, it can lead to nutrient deficiencies, gut dysbiosis, food sensitivities, and even poor immune function.

So, let's see just how well you're absorbing the nutrients from your food and your oxygen! Check any box that applies to you. Each check is one point. Add up your score at the end.

This isn't a diagnosis, it's simply a way to get curious about how your gut may be impacting your energy, mood, hormones, and long-term health.

Core System 1 Questionnaire
Digestive Signs & Symptoms

- ☐ I often feel bloated, full, or gassy after meals.
- ☐ I notice belching, heartburn, or indigestion on a regular basis.
- ☐ I get stomach pain, cramping, or discomfort that doesn't have a clear cause.
- ☐ My bowel habits are inconsistent (constipation, loose stools, or alternating between the two).
- ☐ My stools are unusually large, smelly, oily, or contain undigested food.

- ☐ I've experienced nausea after taking vitamins or supplements.

Immune & Infections

- ☐ I've had recurring yeast or fungal issues (oral thrush, toenail fungus, vaginal yeast infections, athlete's foot, jock itch).
- ☐ I've had chronic gum issues, bleeding gums, or frequent canker sores.
- ☐ I've noticed a whitish coating on my tongue or sore/patchy spots ("geographic tongue").
- ☐ I often have anal or skin itching with no clear cause.

Food & Sensitivities

- ☐ I react to certain foods (bloating, fatigue, rashes, congestion, headaches).
- ☐ Bread, sugar, or refined carbs cause me to feel puffy, foggy, or bloated.
- ☐ I've noticed cravings for sweets, carbs, or alcohol that feel hard to control.

Energy & Mood

- ☐ I feel drained, foggy, or sleepy after eating.
- ☐ I struggle with fatigue that doesn't improve with rest.
- ☐ I notice mood swings, irritability, or anxiety tied to meals or gut issues.

Medications & Stress

- ☐ I've used antibiotics multiple times in the past few years.

- ☐ I've used acid-blocking drugs, antacids, or NSAIDs (ibuprofen, naproxen, aspirin) regularly.
- ☐ I've been on birth control pills, hormone therapy, prednisone, or cortisone.
- ☐ I live under high stress or rarely take time to reset my nervous system.
- ☐ I drink alcohol more than 3 times a week.

Family & Personal History

I or close family members have struggled with:

- ☐ Autoimmune conditions (Hashimoto's, rheumatoid arthritis, lupus, psoriasis, etc.)
- ☐ Chronic skin conditions (eczema, rosacea, adult acne, hives)
- ☐ ADHD, autism spectrum, or other neurodevelopmental challenges
- ☐ Inflammatory bowel conditions (Crohn's, ulcerative colitis, IBS, celiac)
- ☐ Chronic fatigue syndrome or fibromyalgia

> **Your Score:**
>
> <3—Healthy
>
> 4-13—You've got some moderate imbalances—no need to panic. Follow the plan, and let's retest in a month to make sure you're on track!
>
> >14—Severe imbalances—your body's version of sending up a flare. Time to call in the big guns: find a functional medicine practitioner and get the extra testing and support you deserve.

Core System 2: Defense and Repair

Includes: Immune system and inflammation response

Why It's Important:

This system protects the body from infection, clears out damaged cells, and kicks off the healing process. But when it's constantly activated, thanks to chronic inflammation or immune dysfunction, things can go sideways, leading to autoimmune diseases, allergies, or persistent infections.

Our bodies are truly incredible. The sheer amount of work they do, the chemical signaling, and the cell-by-cell repair happening in *each and every cell of our body, every second of every day*, is honestly mind-blowing. Your body is putting in so much effort to keep you going, long before you even notice anything is off.

By the time you feel pain or symptoms, your body has already spent weeks or even months trying to correct the issue quietly behind the scenes. But poor diet and lifestyle choices pile on, and eventually, your body just can't keep up with the inflammation anymore.

The good news? Choosing a healthy lifestyle and diet, even just 80% of the time, gives your body the support it needs to do its job with ease. That includes clearing out those damaged cells we will be talking about in a little while, which in turn helps keep you feeling (and looking) younger. And isn't that the point of it all? Or at least ... one of the big ones.

So, let's see just how many fires we have to put out in your body. Check all that apply to you. This isn't about judgment; it's about connecting the dots between your history, environment, and how your body may be carrying inflammation or stress.

Core System 2 Questionnaire
Immune & Infections

☐ I often catch colds or other infections.

☐ I've dealt with recurring issues like sinus problems, skin rashes, canker sores, or cold sores.

☐ I've had chronic infections in the past (viral, bacterial, or otherwise).

Allergies & Sensitivities

☐ I experience seasonal or environmental allergies.

☐ Certain foods leave me feeling sluggish, foggy, or unwell.

☐ I've had skin reactions such as eczema, acne, or unexplained rashes.

Family Patterns

☐ My family has a history of autoimmune conditions (thyroid issues, rheumatoid arthritis, lupus, etc.).

☐ There's a family history of digestive issues like colitis, irritable bowel, or inflammatory bowel disease.

☐ Alzheimer's, Parkinson's, or other neurodegenerative conditions run in my family.

☐ Heart disease, obesity, or diabetes are common in my family line.

Environment & Exposures

☐ I work or live in a place with poor lighting, limited airflow, or chemical exposure.

☐ I've been exposed to pesticides, heavy metals, or other toxins (including stressful environments or toxic workplaces).

☐ Loud noise, pollution, or other environmental stressors are part of my daily life.

Mind & Mood

☐ I've experienced depression, anxiety, ADHD, or mood swings that feel tied to stress or brain health.

☐ I live a high-stress lifestyle that feels hard to manage.

Body & Lifestyle

☐ I have arthritis, joint pain, or stiffness.

☐ I'm carrying extra weight (BMI over 25) or notice that weight runs in my family.

☐ I exercise for less than 30 minutes, three times per week.

☐ I drink alcohol more than three times a week.

> **Your Score:**
>
> <2—Healthy
>
> 3-10—You've got some moderate imbalances—no need to panic. Follow the plan, and let's retest in a month to make sure you're on track!
>
> >11—Severe imbalances—your body's version of sending up a flare. Time to call in the big guns: find a functional medicine practitioner and get the extra testing and support you deserve.

Core System 3: Energy

Includes: Mitochondrial function, energy production, and metabolism

Why It's Important:

Your body's ability to produce energy, mainly in the form of ATP, is essential for every single cellular process. When that energy production slows down or gets disrupted, you can start feeling fatigued, foggy, slow to recover, and a whole list of metabolic issues no one has time for.

You've probably heard it before, maybe in high school biology or in every health book ever written, that mitochondria are the powerhouse of your cells. But they're not just mini energy plants; they also help regulate what your cells actually do.

Just to put it in some perspective, most cells have hundreds to thousands of mitochondria PER CELL:

- Liver cells have around 1,000–2,000 mitochondria each
- Heart cells have around 5,000 per cell
- A human egg cell has a staggering 100,000 to 600,000
- And at the other end, lymphocytes (white blood cells) have just three

Now think about this: if you've got something like heart disease, that means a significant portion of your mitochondria in those high-energy-demand cells have taken a hit. Considering your body is always working to repair itself, that level of damage didn't happen overnight.

And here's the bigger picture: the more mitochondrial damage you accumulate, the faster your body starts to break down. Cognitively, think increased risk of Parkinson's or Alzheimer's. Metabolically, think diabetes and gut issues, and yes, it all contributes to accelerated aging.

So, let's see just how much fuel you have in your cells. Place a check mark next to any statement that feels true for you. This helps reveal whether your body may be running on "low batteries" from stress, inflammation, or hidden imbalances.

Core System 3 Questionnaire

Energy & Fatigue

- ☐ I experience chronic or long-lasting fatigue.
- ☐ My energy feels drained to the point where daily life feels harder than it should.
- ☐ I often feel exhausted after normal activities or light exercise.
- ☐ Fatigue limits my ability to enjoy hobbies, family time, or work.
- ☐ Sleep doesn't leave me feeling fully refreshed.

Sleep & Recovery

- ☐ I have trouble falling asleep, staying asleep, or waking up too early.
- ☐ Even after a full night of sleep, I feel unrested.
- ☐ My body doesn't bounce back easily after physical or emotional stress.

Body & Physical Health

- ☐ I deal with muscle aches, pain, or unexplained discomfort.
- ☐ I notice muscle weakness or reduced strength.

☐ I've been diagnosed with or suspect conditions like chronic fatigue syndrome or fibromyalgia.

Brain & Mood

☐ I struggle with focus, memory, or mental clarity.

☐ I experience irritability, mood swings, or low resilience under stress.

☐ My symptoms began or worsened after a major stress event, trauma, or infection.

Lifestyle & Environment

☐ I've been exposed to environmental toxins (pesticides, poor-quality water, chemicals, etc.).

☐ I tend to overeat, especially when stressed or fatigued.

☐ I've faced long periods of unrelenting stress.

☐ I've served in high-stress or traumatic environments (such as military combat).

Family & Genetics

☐ Neurological conditions (Alzheimer's, Parkinson's, ALS, etc.) run in my family.

☐ My family has a history of ADHD, autism, or learning differences.

☐ There is a family history of mood disorders such as depression, bipolar disorder, or schizophrenia.

> **Your Score:**
>
> <2—Healthy
>
> 3-10—You've got some moderate imbalances—no need to panic. Follow the plan, and let's retest in a month to make sure you're on track!
>
> >11 —Severe imbalances—your body's version of sending up a flare. Time to call in the big guns: find a functional medicine practitioner and get the extra testing and support you deserve.

Core System 4: Biotransformation and Elimination

Includes: Liver detoxification, kidneys, lungs, skin, lymph

Why It's Important:

OK, this system is seriously amazing. Did you know that you can have up to 70% of your liver removed and it will still grow back to full size? I mean, come on, that's incredibly impressive!

Your intestinal lining replaces itself every three to five days. Your entire blood cell population is recycled and renewed every few weeks. All your body needs is a break and a few better choices every now and then, and it will get to work repairing itself.

This system is responsible for processing and eliminating toxins and waste. But when it gets sluggish or overwhelmed, those toxins can build up, leading to hormonal imbalances, neurological symptoms, and skin issues.

The good news? Your body wants to detox. As long as you're pooping, peeing, sweating, and sleeping, you're clearing out waste and giving your hormones a chance to rebalance.

So, let's see just how toxic you really are. Put a check mark next to any statement that feels true for you. These patterns may point to how well (or not so well) your body is handling daily toxins, environmental stressors, and internal waste removal.

Core System 4 Questionnaire
Elimination & Digestion
- ☐ I often have hard or difficult-to-pass bowel movements.
- ☐ I go to the bathroom every other day (or less frequently).
- ☐ My urine is dark, strong-smelling, or is only produced in small amounts a few times daily.
- ☐ I rarely break a real sweat.

Common Symptoms
- ☐ I deal with one or more of the following:
  - ○ Fatigue
  - ○ Muscle aches
  - ○ Headaches
  - ○ Brain fog or trouble concentrating
- ☐ I have a family history of fibromyalgia or chronic fatigue syndrome.

Lifestyle & Exposures
- ☐ I regularly drink unfiltered tap or well water, or water stored in plastic bottles.

- ☐ I frequently dry-clean my clothes.
- ☐ I spend time in buildings with poor airflow or sealed windows.
- ☐ I live in or near a large city, industrial site, or high-pollution area.
- ☐ I use household, lawn, or pest control chemicals.

Toxin Load & Heavy Metals

- ☐ I have more than one or two silver mercury fillings in my teeth.
- ☐ I eat large fish (tuna, swordfish, shark, tilefish) more than once a week.

Chemical Sensitivities

- ☐ I feel unwell when exposed to strong odors such as:
  - ○ Gasoline or diesel fumes
  - ○ Perfumes or hairspray
  - ○ New car smell or chemical-based cleaners
  - ○ Fabric or dry-cleaning shops
  - ○ Tobacco smoke
  - ○ Chlorinated water

Food & Chemical Reactions

- ☐ I react negatively to foods with preservatives or additives such as MSG, sulfites, sodium benzoate, or artificial ingredients.
- ☐ Even small amounts of alcohol, chocolate, garlic, onions, or aged cheese make me feel unwell.
- ☐ Caffeine leaves me feeling jittery, inflamed, or "crashed out."

Medication & Supplement Use

- ☐ I regularly use medications such as:
  - ○ Pain relievers (Tylenol, ibuprofen, naproxen)
  - ○ Acid blockers or heartburn drugs (Prilosec, Pepcid, Prevacid, etc.)
  - ○ Hormone therapies (birth control, estrogen, progesterone, prostate meds)
  - ○ Allergy, nausea, or digestive symptom medications

Family History & Genetic Susceptibility

- ☐ I've experienced jaundice or been told I have Gilbert's Syndrome.
- ☐ My family has a history of:
  - ○ Breast, prostate, or lung cancer
  - ○ Food sensitivities or allergies
  - ○ Parkinson's, Alzheimer's, ALS, or MS

Your Score:

<2—Healthy

3-10—You've got some moderate imbalances—no need to panic. Follow the plan, and let's retest in a month to make sure you're on track!

>11—Severe imbalances—your body's version of sending up a flare. Time to call in the big guns: find a functional medicine practitioner and get the extra testing and support you deserve.

Core System 5: Communication

Includes: Endocrine (hormones), neurotransmitters, and immune signaling

Why It's Important:

This system is responsible for your body's internal communication, managing everything from hormonal regulation to neurotransmitter balance to immune system coordination.

When it's out of sync, it can show up as mood disorders, thyroid dysfunction, or fertility issues, just to name a few. I'm not going to lie, hormones are complicated. They're sensitive, easily thrown off, and influenced by everything happening in your body. A little too much or too little of anything, and suddenly your whole system is spinning.

As a woman in her 40s, I'll just say it: alcohol hits differently now (you've probably noticed it too … but maybe you're still pretending it doesn't?).

Stress? Hormones hate it.

Diet? Yep, that'll mess them up too.

And don't even get me started on fragrance—put on your favorite perfume and your whole day might unravel. If it doesn't wreck your day, it might just throw off someone else's! Sorry, but you might be unknowingly hormone-bombing your coworkers.

Here's a fun fact: hormones can be measured in picograms per milliliter (pg/mL). A picogram is one trillionth of a gram. That's unbelievably tiny, and yet, when those levels are off? The impact is massive.

So, let's see just how well your hormones are balanced. Place a check mark next to any statement that feels true for you. These patterns may reveal how well your body is handling glucose, insulin, and overall metabolic balance.

Core System 5 Questionnaire

Energy & Mood Swings

- ☐ I crave sweets and often feel an initial "high," followed by a crash.
- ☐ I feel shaky, anxious, or irritable if I go more than a few hours without eating.
- ☐ I notice I get jittery, moody, or headachy throughout the day, but feel better after meals.
- ☐ Missing breakfast (or any meal) makes me cranky, weak, or foggy.
- ☐ Eating makes me feel calm—almost like a "reset button" for my mood.
- ☐ I sometimes get panic or anxiety in the afternoon if I haven't eaten.

Eating Patterns & Triggers

- ☐ If I eat a high-carb breakfast (cereal, bagel, muffin, pancakes), I struggle to control cravings the rest of the day.
- ☐ Once I start eating sweets or carbs, it's hard to stop.
- ☐ I always reach for the bread basket at restaurants.
- ☐ Meals with meat or fish + vegetables help me feel steady, but heavy carb meals (pasta, bread, potatoes, dessert) leave me sleepy or feeling "drugged."

Body & Hormones

- ☐ I carry extra weight around my midsection (waist-to-hip ratio > 0.8).
- ☐ I often feel tired, even after a decent night's sleep.
- ☐ I experience night sweats.
- ☐ My hair is thinning where I want to keep it (scalp) and growing in places it shouldn't (face, chin, etc., if female).
- ☐ I have a history of polycystic ovarian syndrome (PCOS) or infertility.

Symptoms & Signals

- ☐ I get heart palpitations after eating sweets.
- ☐ I seem "salt sensitive" and retain water easily.
- ☐ My memory and concentration aren't as sharp as I'd like.
- ☐ I struggle with irritability, impatience, or low moods.
- ☐ I sometimes feel tired a few hours after eating.

Family History & Susceptibility

- ☐ My family has a history of:
  - Hypoglycemia or blood sugar swings
  - Type 2 diabetes
  - High blood pressure
  - Heart disease
  - Alcoholism
  - Polycystic ovarian syndrome (PCOS)
- ☐ I have a history of chronic fungal or yeast infections (skin, vaginal, jock itch, nail fungus).

> **Your Score:**
>
> <3—Healthy
>
> 4-11—You've got some moderate imbalances—no need to panic. Follow the plan, and let's retest in a month to make sure you're on track!
>
> >12—Severe imbalances—your body's version of sending up a flare. Time to call in the big guns: find a functional medicine practitioner and get the extra testing and support you deserve.

An Additional Test for Women: Sex Hormone Imbalance

Your sex hormones—estrogen, progesterone, and testosterone—are like a three-piece band. When they're in tune, you feel amazing. Your energy is up, your mood is stable, your skin glows, and your weight is stable.

But if one goes off-key, the whole set sounds terrible. That's when you get the mood swings, the PMS from nowhere, the "why am I crying watching animal commercials?" moments. Stress, bad sleep, sugar overload, and even environmental factors can throw the band off.

So what do you do? We need to get all your sex hormones rehearsing together again with good food, movement, stress management, and some TLC. Once they're back in harmony, you'll feel like yourself again in no time.

Place a check mark by any statement that feels true for you. These patterns can reveal how your hormones may be talking to you and where your body might be asking for extra support.

Monthly Cycle & PMS

☐ I experience premenstrual symptoms (irritability, bloating, cramps, mood swings, etc.).
☐ My weight fluctuates noticeably throughout my cycle.
☐ I deal with swelling, puffiness, or water retention.
☐ I often feel bloated before or during my period.
☐ I get headaches or migraines around my cycle.
☐ I have strong premenstrual cravings (especially sugar or salty foods).
☐ I feel emotionally low, irritable, or unable to cope with everyday demands during my cycle.
☐ My breasts become swollen, tender, or lumpy before my period.

Fertility & Reproductive Health

☐ My cycle is irregular, with heavy or very light bleeding.
☐ I've struggled with infertility.
☐ I have a history of breast cysts, fibrocystic breasts, or uterine fibroids.
☐ I use birth control pills or other synthetic hormones.
☐ I have a family history of breast, ovarian, or uterine cancer.
☐ I have a family history of fibroids or hormone-related conditions.

Perimenopause & Menopause

☐ I experience hot flashes or night sweats.
☐ I have trouble sleeping (falling asleep, staying asleep, or waking too early).

- ☐ My sex drive has declined.
- ☐ I notice dryness of the skin, hair, or vagina.
- ☐ I feel anxious, irritable, or moody.
- ☐ I've noticed new or worsening heart palpitations.
- ☐ My memory or concentration feels foggy.
- ☐ I've gained weight—especially around my middle.
- ☐ I've noticed unwanted facial hair growth.

Environment & Lifestyle

- ☐ I've been exposed to pesticides, heavy metals, or other environmental toxins (through food, water, air, or chemicals).

Your Score:

<3—Healthy

4-12—You've got some moderate imbalances—no need to panic. Follow the plan, and let's retest in a month to make sure you're on track!

>13—Severe imbalances—your body's version of sending up a flare. Time to call in the big guns: find a functional medicine practitioner and get the extra testing and support you deserve.

An Additional Test for Men: Sex Hormone Imbalance

Your male hormones (mainly testosterone, but a few others are in the mix) are like your body's head coach. When the coach is calling great plays, you've got energy, drive, muscle, focus, and you're feeling on top of your game.

But if the coach gets tired, distracted, or benched, you will experience low energy, brain fog, muscle loss, stubborn belly fat, and a "meh" mood. Stress, lack of sleep, poor diet, too much alcohol, and even everyday chemicals can take the coach out of the game.

Enter lifestyle changes, strength training, quality sleep, better nutrition, and managing stress, and you can get the coach back on the field and your whole team playing like champions again.

Place a check next to any statement that feels true for you. This self-check isn't about judgment; it's about noticing where your body and mind may be signaling the need for support.

Energy, Drive & Mood

- ☐ My sex drive has noticeably declined.
- ☐ I feel less vitality and motivation than I used to.
- ☐ I often feel apathetic, directionless, or lacking purpose.
- ☐ I experience frequent fatigue or low energy.
- ☐ My mood tends to be low, irritable, or flat.

Reproductive & Sexual Health

- ☐ I have difficulty achieving or maintaining an erection.
- ☐ I've been told I have (or suspect) a low sperm count.
- ☐ I've struggled with infertility.

Strength & Body Composition

- ☐ I've noticed muscle loss or reduced strength.
- ☐ My belly fat has increased (especially around the abdomen).
- ☐ I feel physically weaker than I used to.
- ☐ I've experienced bone thinning or even fractures.

Family & Lifestyle Factors

- ☐ I have a family history of high cholesterol.
- ☐ I have a family history of insulin resistance, diabetes, or blood sugar issues.
- ☐ I've been exposed to pesticides, heavy metals, or environmental toxins.

> **Your Score:**
>
> <2—Healthy
>
> 3-7—You've got some moderate imbalances—no need to panic. Follow the plan, and let's retest in a month to make sure you're on track!
>
> >8—Severe imbalances—your body's version of sending up a flare. Time to call in the big guns: find a functional medicine practitioner and get the extra testing and support you deserve.

Thyroid Imbalance

From a functional medicine perspective, a thyroid imbalance isn't just a "thyroid problem," it's a signal that your whole system needs attention. Your thyroid is like your body's thermostat, controlling energy, metabolism, mood, and even hair and skin health.

When it's off, whether running too slow or too fast, it's often tied to deeper issues like nutrient deficiencies, chronic stress, inflammation, gut imbalances, or even hidden toxins.

Instead of just turning the thermostat up or down with medication, functional medicine looks for *why* it's misreading the temperature in the first place so you can restore balance from the ground up.

Put a check mark next to any statements that feel true for you. These clues may point to how your thyroid and the hormones it regulates are impacting your energy, metabolism, and overall well-being.

Skin, Hair & Nails

- ☐ My skin feels thick or unusually dry.
- ☐ My hair is thinning, coarse, or shedding more than usual.
- ☐ My fingernails are thick or brittle.
- ☐ The outer third of my eyebrows seems to be thinning.

Temperature & Circulation

- ☐ I'm sensitive to cold.
- ☐ My hands and feet are often cold.
- ☐ I retain fluids (swelling in hands, feet, or puffiness).
- ☐ I sweat less than most people.

Energy & Muscles

- ☐ I wake up feeling tired or sluggish, even after a full night's sleep.
- ☐ I experience muscle fatigue, aches, or weakness.
- ☐ My blood pressure and/or heart rate tend to run low.

Weight, Digestion & Metabolism

- ☐ I've gained weight recently or struggle to lose weight despite healthy efforts.
- ☐ I experience constipation regularly.

☐ My appetite and metabolism feel slower than they used to.

Hormones & Reproductive Health

☐ My sex drive has decreased.

☐ I have heavy periods, worsening PMS, or fertility challenges.

Mood & Cognition

☐ I have difficulty with memory, focus, or concentration.

☐ My mood feels flat, apathetic, or low.

Family & Environmental Factors

☐ I have a family history of thyroid problems.

☐ I have a family history of autoimmune disease (rheumatoid arthritis, lupus, MS, celiac, allergies, yeast overgrowth).

☐ I've been exposed to radiation or environmental toxins.

☐ I consume a lot of tuna/sushi or have multiple dental silver (mercury) fillings.

☐ I drink chlorinated or fluoridated tap water.

Your Score:

<3—Healthy

4-11—You've got some moderate imbalances—no need to panic. Follow the plan, and let's retest in a month to make sure you're on track!

>12—Severe imbalances—your body's version of sending up a flare. Time to call in the big guns: find a functional medicine practitioner and get the extra testing and support you deserve.

Core System 6: Transport

Includes: Cardiovascular and lymphatic systems

Why It's Important:

OK, I want you to really understand just how important your cardiovascular and lymphatic systems are. These are your body's transport networks that move nutrients, hormones, immune cells, and waste products. When they slow down or break down, so do you.

Cardiovascular System

Your heart beats about 100,000 times a day. That's around 35 million beats a year, with no days off, and it's only the size of your fist. It pumps around 1.5 gallons (five to six liters) of blood per minute, adding up to 2,000 gallons (7,500 liters) daily, enough to fill a small swimming pool. It pushes blood through 60,000 miles of blood vessels, which is enough to wrap around the Earth twice. In under a minute, it delivers blood to every cell in your body.

Exercise strengthens your heart muscle, which is why (spoiler alert) you'll hear about exercise throughout this whole book. Your only limit will ever be *you*. Walking, dancing, swimming, and even chasing your kids or your dog all help your heart pump more efficiently.

During intense activity, your heart can increase output up to seven times, going from a resting five liters per minute to over 25–35 liters in elite athletes.

Lymphatic System

This is your body's drainage and detox crew, collecting waste, toxins, excess fluid, and dead cells and moving them out. It's also essential for your immune system. You've got 600–700 lymph nodes, mostly in your neck, armpits, abdomen, and groin, constantly scanning for invaders.

If your lymphatic system gets sluggish, so does your immunity. Unlike your cardiovascular system, there's no pump here. Lymph depends on movement, so walking, stretching, deep breathing, and even jumping all help it flow (yep, exercise shows up again!). Fun fact: you have about twice as much lymph as blood quietly doing its job in the background.

So yes, if these systems aren't running well, it's game over for efficient transport. You'll see a breakdown in everything from nutrient delivery and immune defense to waste removal, and that can show up as inflammation, swelling, fatigue, and chronic disease. Keep them moving, and you stay moving.

Let's see just how well your blood reaches the tips of your fingers and ends of your toes and comes back around!

Place a check mark next to any statement that rings true for you. Your circulation is the lifeline of your body, delivering oxygen, nutrients, and healing signals everywhere. These questions help reveal where your heart and blood vessels may need extra support.

Core System 6 Questionnaire
Heart & Blood Pressure

- ☐ I've been diagnosed with heart disease (angina or a past heart attack).
- ☐ I have high blood pressure.
- ☐ I experience poor circulation, especially in my feet.

Fluid Balance & Swelling

☐ My hands and/or feet often swell.

☐ I notice edema (fluid retention or puffiness).

Blood Flow & Vitality

☐ I experience erectile dysfunction.

☐ I get muscle cramps.

☐ My hands and feet often feel cold.

☐ I've been diagnosed with Raynaud's syndrome (fingers or toes turn white or blue in the cold).

Immune & Healing

☐ I get frequent infections.

☐ My wounds heal slowly.

Vascular Clues

☐ I have varicose veins.

☐ I've experienced blood clots.

☐ I notice tingling, numbness, or "pins and needles" in my arms, hands, legs, or feet.

Your Score:

<2—Healthy

3–7—You've got some moderate imbalances—no need to panic. Follow the plan, and let's retest in a month to make sure you're on track!

> **>8**—Severe imbalances—your body's version of sending up a flare. Time to call in the big guns: find a functional medicine practitioner and get the extra testing and support you deserve.

Core System 7: Structural Integrity

Includes: Musculoskeletal system, cell membranes, and extracellular matrix

Why It's Important:

The body's structure is what holds everything together, literally! It plays a huge role in how well everything functions. When structural integrity is compromised, it can lead to chronic pain, injuries, mobility issues, and even dysfunction at the cellular level, particularly around cell membranes.

Just a reminder: your body is constantly working behind the scenes to fix things and manage inflammation, but when it gets overloaded, the first signal it sends you is usually pain.

Of course, there's more to it—stress, poor nutrition, your life stage, and even socio-economic factors—but one of the most common (and overlooked) culprits in poor structural health is posture, posture, posture!

There's also growing research showing connections between posture and neurodevelopmental conditions like ADHD, ADD, and autism, especially when we consider how posture reflects and affects nervous system function, sensory processing, and motor control.

Now, to be clear, posture doesn't cause these conditions, but it can definitely influence how they show up. A huge part of posture is core strength, especially around the spine and pelvis. Strong core muscles help you sit, stand, and move efficiently. So *exercise!*

But if core stability is weak in kids or adults, it's harder to sit upright for long periods. That slouched, slumped-over position? It can reduce blood flow to the brain and make it harder to stay focused, alert, and attentive, all things that are already challenging in ADHD and ADD.

Poor posture can also reflect problems with proprioception (your ability to sense where your body is in space), which can lead to clumsiness, weird sitting positions, or just feeling uncomfortable in your own body.

So, let's see just how well your body is holding you together! Put a check mark next to any statement that applies to you. Muscles aren't just for athletes; they're your body's longevity reserve. They protect your bones, stabilize your joints, regulate blood sugar, and keep your metabolism humming.

Core System 7 Questionnaire
Strength & Daily Function
- ☐ I've lost noticeable muscle mass over the years.
- ☐ I find it harder to do daily tasks that require strength (lifting groceries, climbing stairs, opening jars).
- ☐ I don't currently do strength or resistance training.

Diet & Protein Intake
- ☐ I follow a vegan or vegetarian diet.

☐ I eat less than 25–30 grams of protein per meal.
☐ I don't eat fish or take omega-3 fatty acid supplements.
☐ I eat fried or ultra-processed foods often.

Bone & Energy Support

☐ I've been diagnosed with osteopenia or osteoporosis.
☐ I don't take vitamin D3 supplements.
☐ I often experience low energy or stamina.

> **Your Score:**
>
> <1—Healthy
>
> 2-5—You've got some moderate imbalances—no need to panic. Follow the plan, and let's retest in a month to make sure you're on track!
>
> >6— Severe imbalances—your body's version of sending up a flare. Time to call in the big guns: find a functional medicine practitioner and get the extra testing and support you deserve.

Essential Fatty Acids Deficiency (Omega-3s)

An essential fatty acid deficiency is like trying to run a car without enough oil; things start to squeak, slow down, and wear out faster. These healthy fats, especially omega-3s, 6s, 7s, and 9s, are critical for brain health, hormone balance, reducing inflammation, keeping your skin supple, and supporting your mood.

One of the best ways to measure your levels is with the Omega-3 Index, a blood test that shows how much omega-3 is in your red blood cells. We want it above 4%, but optimal is between 8–10% to significantly lower your risk of heart disease, Alzheimer's, and other inflammation-driven conditions.

When you're low, you might notice dry skin, joint pain, fatigue, brain fog, or even more intense PMS symptoms. Instead of just patching the squeaks, we look at *why* you're low, whether it's diet, digestion, or absorption. That way, we can make sure you're getting and using these fats so your body runs smoothly for the long haul.

Check off any statements that apply to you. Essential fatty acids (EFAs) are called *essential* for a reason; your body can't make them on its own. They're critical for healthy skin, flexible joints, sharp memory, balanced hormones, and even mood stability. When you're running low, your body starts sending signals, sometimes in sneaky ways.

Skin, Hair & Nails

- ☐ My nails are soft, cracked, or brittle.
- ☐ My skin feels dry, itchy, flaky, or scaly.
- ☐ I get "chicken skin" (tiny bumps on the back of my arms or torso).
- ☐ I have dandruff or a flaky scalp.
- ☐ My earwax tends to be hard or dry.

Joints, Gut & Hydration

- ☐ I often feel achy or stiff in my joints.
- ☐ I'm thirsty most of the time.
- ☐ I struggle with constipation (fewer than two bowel movements per day).

☐ My stools are light-colored, hard, or foul-smelling.

Brain, Mood & Hormones

☐ I experience low mood, poor focus, or memory lapses.
☐ I have high blood pressure.
☐ I've been told I have fibrocystic breasts.
☐ I notice PMS symptoms regularly.

Family & Ancestry Clues

☐ My family history includes high LDL cholesterol, low HDL, or high triglycerides.

☐ I have a North Atlantic genetic background (Irish, Scottish, Welsh, Scandinavian, or coastal Native American)—groups more prone to essential fatty acid imbalances.

> **Your Score:**
>
> <2—Healthy
>
> 3-7—You've got some moderate imbalances—no need to panic. Follow the plan, and let's retest in a month to make sure you're on track!
>
> >8—Severe imbalances—your body's version of sending up a flare. Time to call in the big guns: find a functional medicine practitioner and get the extra testing and support you deserve.

Vitamin D Deficiency

Vitamin D deficiency isn't just about weak bones; it's like running your immune system, brain, and hormones on low battery.

Vitamin D acts more like a hormone than a vitamin, influencing everything from mood and energy to inflammation and immune defense.

Low levels are linked to higher risks of heart disease, depression, autoimmune conditions, and even certain cancers. We measure it with a simple blood test, and while anything above 30 ng/mL is considered "normal," optimal wellness lives between 50–80 ng/mL.

In some autoimmune diseases, we would even prefer to see the levels closer to 100ng/mL. If you're low, we don't just hand you a supplement; we look at why. Is it a lack of sun, poor absorption, gut issues, or chronic inflammation?

Place a check next to any that apply to you. Because so many of us spend our days indoors, Vitamin D deficiencies are incredibly common (even in sunny places!). Let's see if your body is waving some red flags.

Mood & Cognitive Health

- ☐ My family has a history of seasonal affective disorder (SAD) or winter blues.
- ☐ I've noticed a loss of mental sharpness or memory.

Bones & Muscles

- ☐ My muscles often feel sore or weak.
- ☐ My bones feel tender when pressed (like on the shin).
- ☐ I have osteoarthritis.
- ☐ I've broken more than two bones or have had a hip fracture.
- ☐ My family has a history of osteoporosis.

Sunlight & Lifestyle Habits

- ☐ I work indoors most of the time.
- ☐ I avoid direct sunlight or wear sunscreen nearly every day.
- ☐ I live north of Florida (less direct sunlight throughout the year).

Food & Nutrient Sources

- ☐ I don't regularly eat small fatty fish (sardines, mackerel, herring).
- ☐ My family has a history of autoimmune conditions (such as MS).
- ☐ My family has a history of prostate cancer.

Skin Color & Age Factors

- ☐ I have darker skin (melanin reduces vitamin D production).
- ☐ I'm age 60 or older.

Your Score:

<2—Healthy

3-7—You've got some moderate imbalances—no need to panic. Follow the plan, and let's retest in a month to make sure you're on track!

>8—Severe imbalances—your body's version of sending up a flare. Time to call in the big guns: find a functional medicine practitioner and get the extra testing and support you deserve.

Magnesium Deficiency

Magnesium deficiency is like pulling the spark plugs out of your body's engine. Things might still run, but not smoothly. Magnesium is involved in over 300 biochemical reactions, including muscle function, nerve signaling, blood sugar control, sleep regulation, and stress response.

Low magnesium can show up as muscle cramps, headaches, anxiety, poor sleep, heart palpitations, or constipation. We like to look beyond blood tests because magnesium lives mostly inside your cells, not floating around in your bloodstream.

If you're low, we dig into why—stress, poor diet, gut malabsorption, and certain medications could be the culprits—and then restore it with magnesium-rich foods or targeted supplementation so your body can fire on all cylinders again.

Place a check mark by any statement that feels true for you. Magnesium is often called the "master mineral," yet most people are walking around deficient, and the symptoms can show up everywhere from mood to muscles to metabolism.

Mood & Mind

☐ I often feel low, irritable, or anxious.
☐ I struggle with focus or concentration.
☐ I have trouble falling or staying asleep.
☐ I'm sensitive to loud noises.
☐ I get frequent headaches or migraines.

Muscles & Movement

- ☐ I notice twitching in my muscles.
- ☐ I have leg or hand cramps.
- ☐ I experience restless legs, especially at night.
- ☐ I feel fatigued even when I get enough rest.
- ☐ I suffer from constipation (fewer than two bowel movements per day).

Heart & Nervous System

- ☐ I've experienced heart flutters, skipped beats, or palpitations.
- ☐ I have a family history of heart disease, heart failure, or mitral valve prolapse.
- ☐ I have acid reflux or trouble swallowing.

Hormones & Other Clues

- ☐ I experience premenstrual syndrome (PMS).
- ☐ I've been under excessive stress for long periods.
- ☐ I have kidney stones.

Family & Nutrition

- ☐ I have a family history of asthma, autism, or diabetes.
- ☐ My diet is low in magnesium-rich foods such as kelp, wheat bran, almonds, cashews, or dark leafy greens.

> **Your Score:**
>
> <2—Healthy
>
> 3-9—You've got some moderate imbalances—no need to panic. Follow the plan, and let's retest in a month to make sure you're on track!
>
> >10—Severe imbalances—your body's version of sending up a flare. Time to call in the big guns: find a functional medicine practitioner and get the extra testing and support you deserve.

Zinc Deficiency

Zinc deficiency is like taking the security team out of your body's headquarters; suddenly, the doors are wide open for trouble. Zinc is essential for immune defense, wound healing, hormone production, skin health, taste and smell, and even brain function.

Low zinc can show up as frequent colds, slow healing cuts, hair loss, brittle nails, changes in taste or smell, acne, or hormonal imbalances. We also look at copper balance, because too much copper can block zinc's effectiveness.

If you're low on zinc, the goal isn't just to pop a supplement; we check diet, gut health, and possible medication interactions so zinc can actually do its job as your body's microscopic security guard.

Place a check mark by the statements that feel true for you. Zinc is one of the most underrated minerals, yet it influences everything from your sense of taste and smell to immune strength, hormone balance, and skin health.

Senses & Signals

- ☐ My sense of taste feels dulled.
- ☐ My sense of smell seems impaired.
- ☐ My nails are weak, thin, brittle, or peeling.
- ☐ I notice white spots on my nails.

Immune & Infections

- ☐ I get frequent colds or respiratory infections.
- ☐ I deal with allergies often.
- ☐ My wounds take a long time to heal.
- ☐ I experience diarrhea.

Skin & Hair

- ☐ I have eczema or other rashes.
- ☐ I struggle with acne.
- ☐ I have dandruff.
- ☐ I am experiencing hair loss.

Hormones & Reproductive Health

- ☐ I have a family history of erectile dysfunction.
- ☐ I have an enlarged or inflamed prostate.
- ☐ I have a family history of rheumatoid arthritis or inflammatory bowel disease (ulcerative colitis, Crohn's).

Lifestyle & Risk Factors

- ☐ I drink hard water (which can interfere with zinc absorption).
- ☐ I consume more than three alcoholic drinks per week.

- ☐ I sweat excessively (sports, sauna, or high stress).
- ☐ I use diuretics (water pills).
- ☐ I am over the age of 65.

Nutrition & Intake

- ☐ My diet is low in zinc-rich foods such as dulse (seaweed), fresh ginger root, egg yolks, fish, lamb, legumes, pumpkin seeds, or kelp.

> **Your Score:**
>
> <2—Healthy
>
> 3-11—You've got some moderate imbalances—no need to panic. Follow the plan, and let's retest in a month to make sure you're on track!
>
> >12—Severe imbalances—your body's version of sending up a flare. Time to call in the big guns: find a functional medicine practitioner and get the extra testing and support you deserve.

Methylation Imbalance

Methylation is like your body's master multitasking app. It's quietly running in the background, controlling everything from detox and DNA repair to brain chemistry, hormone balance, and immune function.

If methylation isn't working well, you might notice fatigue, mood changes, poor detox tolerance, inflammation, or faster signs of aging. We can check methylation status through specific functional lab markers, including certain B-vitamin levels and homocysteine. Optimal methylation helps your body turn nutrients into active compounds, turns genes on or off as needed, and keeps inflammation in check.

If it's sluggish, we look at nutrition (especially folate, B12, and B6), lifestyle stressors, and toxin exposure. I'll walk you through this in more detail later, but for now, think of it as one of your body's most important "behind-the-scenes" systems for staying healthy and resilient.

Put a check mark by each statement that applies to you. Folate (a B vitamin found mostly in leafy greens) and your body's ability to methylate (turn nutrients into active forms your cells can use) play a huge role in mood, memory, energy, and even how you age.

Diet & Lifestyle

- ☐ I eat animal protein (meat, dairy, cheese, eggs) more than 5 times per week.
- ☐ My portions of animal protein are usually larger than the size of my palm (4–6 oz).
- ☐ I eat processed or packaged foods that contain hydrogenated oils or shortening more than once per week.
- ☐ I eat fewer than 1 cup of leafy greens daily.
- ☐ I eat fewer than 5–9 servings of fruits and vegetables per day.
- ☐ I drink more than 3 alcoholic beverages per week.
- ☐ I don't currently take a multivitamin.

Mood & Cognitive Function

- ☐ I struggle with low mood.

- ☐ I have noticed memory issues, balance problems, or tingling in my feet.
- ☐ I have a family or personal history of dementia, Alzheimer's, or other cognitive decline.
- ☐ I have been diagnosed with MS, neuropathy, or nerve-related issues (like carpal tunnel).

Cardiovascular & Cancer Risk

- ☐ I have had a heart attack or been diagnosed with heart disease.
- ☐ I have had a stroke or circulation issues.
- ☐ I have a history of cancer (colon, cervical, breast, or other).
- ☐ I am over 65 years old.

Reproductive Health

- ☐ I have a history of abnormal PAP tests.
- ☐ I have a history of birth defects in offspring (neural tube defects, Down syndrome, etc.).

Your Score:

<2—Healthy

3-9—You've got some moderate imbalances—no need to panic. Follow the plan, and let's retest in a month to make sure you're on track!

>10—Severe imbalances—your body's version of sending up a flare. Time to call in the big guns: find a functional medicine practitioner and get the extra testing and support you deserve.

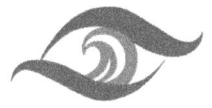

Age Is Just a Number— But Which One?

Now that you've done a little systemic self-inspection (go you!), I hope it's made a few light bulbs go off about which areas of your body need some extra love and attention.

If you're freaking out a little or feeling discouraged, don't. Seriously, in just 10 short days, you can start lowering inflammation, boosting your energy, losing weight, and reducing chronic disease symptoms by up to 70%. That's huge!

Which brings us to the next topic . . . your biological age.

Biological Age vs. Chronological Age

Chronological age: how many candles are on your birthday cake.

Biological age: how old your body actually feels and functions based on your health.

Two people can be 40 years old, but one has the energy and vitality of a 30-year-old, and the other feels 60. What's the difference? Diet, movement, stress, sleep, inflammation, and lifestyle habits.

The good news? You can change your biological age starting at *any* age. This is what we call preventative work, and it's powerful.

Let me tell you a story. My younger brother constantly reminds me not to "sweat the small stuff" and to stop worrying about things that haven't happened. (Yes, I've read *Don't Sweat the Small Stuff* by Richard Carlson, and yes, I still sweat the small stuff sometimes.)

But here's the thing, your health doesn't need your stress; it needs your attention. Build smart, healthy habits now, and you'll spend far less time worrying later.

Remember: "Prevention is better than cure," my dad's all-time favorite quote. I have spent a lifetime listening to him say it, in all aspects of my life: health, finances, the type of friends I choose, and the schools I picked. Everything can be prevented if I think before I act, according to him! (For better or worse, he is right.)

> "If you don't make time for your health,
> you'll be forced to make time for your illness."

> "If you don't invest in your health now,
> you'll end up investing in disease later."[1]

Let's talk money for a second. Keeping yourself healthy may cost an estimated $250,000 to $500,000+ over your lifetime ($3,000–$7,000/year on wellness, food, supplements, movement, etc.).

---

[1] 1. Martin Meadows, *Daily Self-Discipline: Everyday Habits and Exercises to Build Self-Discipline and Achieve Your Goals* (Lulu Press, 2018).

Before you say, "That's a lot!" think about how many people spend $5 a day on Starbucks. That's $500–$600 a year just on coffee that may actually create inflammation. Unless it's organic, mold-free, third-party tested (which, let's be real, it usually isn't), that cup might be adding to your toxic load.

And we don't just spend money on coffee; how often do we hit "Buy Now" on Amazon without thinking? (Guilty!) So yes, most people do have the money, it's just not going toward their health until they're forced to.

Now let's talk about what happens when you choose to ignore all the preventative stuff:

$1,000,000–$3,000,000+ is what chronic illness can cost over a lifetime. We're talking heart disease, diabetes, Alzheimer's, autoimmune diseases, cancer, and the list goes on. It's not just expensive; it drastically lowers your quality of life.

Let me break it down for you one more time:

Chronological age = How long you've been alive. Biological age = How well your body is aging internally based on:

- Nutrition
- Movement
- Sleep
- Stress
- Toxins
- Genetic expression (hello, epigenetics!)

This is why your healthspan matters.

Ok, so let's talk lifespan vs. healthspan vs. sickspan.

- Lifespan: Total years you live from birth to death
- Healthspan: Years you live without chronic disease or disability
- Sickspan: The part where you're alive, but sick, tired, or just getting by

Your goal should be to maximize your healthspan and minimize that dreaded sickspan. With the tools in this book and companion resources available on my website, you can start turning back your biological clock at ANY age. That's the beauty of the human body. It wants to heal. You just have to give it a chance.

Also, let's clear something up. One of my biggest pet peeves is when a doctor says, "Oh, that's normal for your age." OMG, I swear I want to scream. That and when people don't use their indicators when they drive, at least here in California . . . I mean, seriously, I just don't get it. It's not bling, bling on your car; it tells the people around you what you are planning on doing so that they know to either slow down or stop. OK, I digress.

Just because something occurs often in many people does NOT mean that it's normal. It simply means that we don't know the solution or are not trying to find one.

Common Aging vs. Optimal Aging

- Common aging: Things start breaking down. You hurt. You get chronic or terminal diseases.
- Optimal aging: You function across the board physically, emotionally, cognitively, socially, and spiritually without disease. Then you go to sleep one day and never wake up!.

Here's the curveball: The World Health Organization actually classifies aging as a disease. The U.S. medical system doesn't ... yet. But think about it, if smoking increases cancer risk 5x and aging increases it 50x, then aging is a disease.

Now, let's get a little nerdy (but in a fun way).

Why Do We Age?

Our cells are constantly renewing, especially in the gut, skin, lungs, immune system, and even parts of the brain (like the hippocampus, which handles learning and memory). Stem cells play a key role here because they can turn into anything your body needs.

If our cells are constantly renewing, how do we age?

Over time, due to poor diet, stress, toxins, and inactivity, these cells weaken. Eventually, our cells stop dividing and go into what we call senescence; in other words, they get old and cranky. Senescent cells are troublemakers. They leak inflammation, send confusing signals, and drag down the healthy cells around them.

Imagine a bowl of fresh, shiny, beautiful fruit. Each piece represents a healthy cell in your body. Now, picture a single lemon in the middle starting to rot. Not only does that lemon become inedible, but the rot begins to spread to the nearby fruit touching it.

That's exactly what happens with senescent cells in your body when they stop functioning properly. They don't just sit quietly; they affect the healthy cells around them, spreading dysfunction and inflammation like that rotting lemon. The key to staying young and vibrant is to keep your cells healthy and renewing properly. That's what this book is here to help you do.

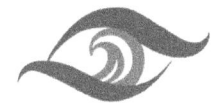

The Blue Zones

Imagine living to 100 years old with no health problems and feeling full of energy. You walk your neighborhood with ease, tend to your garden, your memory is sharp enough to recall your favorite childhood stories, and you're not taking a single medication.

Sounds dreamy, right? By now, you've probably heard of the five Blue Zones around the world. There are books on them, and Netflix even has a whole show, definitely worth watching!

These are regions where an unusually high number of people live to 100+ while staying active, engaged, and healthy in their communities. Drum roll, please ...

- Sardinia, Italy
- Okinawa, Japan
- Ikaria, Greece
- Nicoya, Costa Rica
- Loma Linda, California

These communities have 20 times the number of centenarians compared to the U.S. After studying them, researchers discovered that these long-living populations share five key lifestyle habits:

- Diet
- Movement
- Strong family and community ties
- Purpose
- Minimal stress

Let's Talk Diet

The Japanese have a saying: "Hara Hachi Bun Me." It's a Confucian teaching that means "eat until you're 80% full." The idea is simple: stop eating before you feel stuffed. Many centenarians grow and/or hunt their own food.

Now, I'm not suggesting you buy a gun or a spear and head into the wilderness, but you can support this mindset by shopping from local farmers, choosing seasonal produce, and buying animal products from sources that treat and harvest animals humanely. Also, they do not eat anything imported or artificial.

Their diets are high in:

- Vegetables—full of fiber, vitamins, and minerals that significantly lower the risk of heart disease and cancer.
- Legumes—rich in fiber and protein, and associated with lower mortality rates.
- Whole grains—great for reducing blood pressure and lowering the risk of heart disease and colorectal cancer.

- Nuts—high in fiber, healthy fats, and protein; they support long-term health and longevity.
- Meat—when consumed, it's usually from animals they raise themselves. They often say they "flavor the meat before they kill the animal," meaning the animal eats a phytochemical-rich diet. They also consume the whole animal, including organ meats, which are incredibly nutrient-dense (we'll get more into this later!).

Here's something powerful: a study published in *The Journal of the American Medical Association* found that starting a Mediterranean diet and walking regimen at age 70 reduced the risk of death by a whopping 60%.[2] That's the fork in the road I mentioned earlier; it's never too late to choose health.

And yes, yet another mouse study, but this one's wild. In this experiment, mice were given a single high-glucose meal. The study only lasted six days, but that one sugary meal had lasting effects. It changed how the DNA in vascular (blood vessel) cells expressed themselves, increasing free radical production (bad) and suppressing antioxidant genes (also bad). So just one high-sugar meal disrupted the body's balance for more than six days.[3] Mic. Drop.

---

[2] Knoops KT;de Groot LC;Kromhout D;Perrin AE;Moreiras-Varela O;Menotti A;van Staveren WA;, "Mediterranean Diet, Lifestyle Factors, and 10-Year Mortality in Elderly European Men and Women: The Hale Project," JAMA, accessed August 12, 2025, https://pubmed.ncbi.nlm.nih.gov/15383513/.

[3] Marpadga A Reddy and Rama Natarajan, "Epigenetic Mechanisms in Diabetic Vascular Complications," Cardiovascular research, June 1, 2011, https://pmc.ncbi.nlm.nih.gov/articles/PMC3096305/?utm_source=chatgpt.com.

Again, I'm not telling you this to shame you, but to empower you. If you love fast food and soda, that's your call. You can stick with that lifestyle and see how far you get before your body starts waving the white flag. But maybe today, you decide to give up fast food while still keeping your soda. That, in itself, is a huge win.

Want to know the quickest way to fail? Try to change everything at once. Instead, just pick one bad habit and remove it from your life for 21–28 days. Once that's solid, pick the next.

One step at a time, and you will succeed. Think of it like driving from Spain to Croatia at night. You only need to see the next 200 feet in front of you, thanks to your headlights, then the next 200 feet and then the next. That's how you get across Europe, step by step.

Let's Talk Movement

Movement doesn't have to mean going to the gym and lifting weights. It simply means don't be stagnant.

Objects in motion stay in motion. Objects at rest . . . well, you know the rest.

The Japanese often sit on the floor, which naturally keeps them flexible and mobile. This full range of motion, used every day, helps prevent joint issues. Compare that to most Westerners, who sit in chairs all day with very limited joint engagement.

Movement comes in many forms: walking, dancing, gardening, tai chi—all are wonderful for your body and mind.

Here's something cool: walking barefoot or playing in the dirt is incredibly good for you. Not only do you move and socialize, but you're also grounding yourself. The Earth is full of negative ions (the good kind), which help reduce inflammation and calm the nervous system. On the flip side, the air around us, especially indoors, is loaded with positive ions, which can increase anxiety and inflammation.

Grounding (also called "earthing") has been shown to:

- Reduce white blood cell counts (linked to inflammation)
- Increase red blood cells (boosting oxygen and immunity)
- Improve sleep
- Increase antioxidants
- Support balance and proprioception
- Strengthen joints, ligaments, and muscles in your lower body

Exercise also dramatically reduces the risk of heart disease, cancer, diabetes, and early death. Those who age well build movement into their daily lives. People who maintain a healthy weight, don't smoke, and move regularly tend to live long, vibrant lives, and when the time comes, they often pass quickly and peacefully. Those who don't? Their final years can be long, painful, and expensive. Harsh truth, but truth nonetheless.

Let's Talk Family & Community

You've probably heard about studies where monkeys kept in isolation showed severe developmental delays or about children around the world who were locked away and isolated, resulting in permanent developmental harm. Isolation can affect us at any age, and its consequences are serious.

Loneliness and social isolation have been linked to many health issues, including:

- Heart disease and stroke
- Type 2 diabetes
- Depression and anxiety
- Suicide and self-harm
- Addiction
- Cognitive decline
- Dementia and even early death

But did you know there's a difference between social isolation and loneliness?

Social isolation means having very few or no social contacts or relationships. Even if someone doesn't feel lonely, this lack of connection still puts them at risk for these health problems.

Loneliness, on the other hand, is the feeling of being disconnected or alone, even if you have many friends around you. It's the sense that you lack meaningful relationships or a true sense of belonging.

So far, we've talked about diet, exercise, and movement as keys to living a long and healthy life. But the people living longest and healthiest also share something else incredibly important: a strong sense of community, family, and belonging.

They cook and eat together, walk and move together, tell stories, laugh, and socialize across all ages. The young and old mix freely throughout their days and nights. Everyone talks, and everyone listens.

If you don't have a close blood family or if your relationships aren't supportive, it's okay, you can create your own community, your own family. This is truly that important. Laughter really is the best medicine, and it's always better shared with others.

Not everyone is fortunate enough to have a kind, loving, or close family or friend group. Sometimes, the people around us can even add stress or accelerate aging. But here's the good news: you have the power to choose your friends and family.

I encourage you to choose the ones who uplift you, support you, and help you age in reverse. Family and community aren't just nice-to-haves; they're essential for thriving and living a vibrant, long life.

Let's Talk Purpose

The science is clear: people who have a strong sense of purpose tend to live longer, regardless of their lifestyle habits. Now, that's not a free pass to find your purpose and hit the McDonald's drive-thru three times a day, but it does highlight just how powerful purpose really is.

What exactly is purpose? While it looks different for everyone, at its core, purpose means having a reason to get up in the morning, a goal or direction that gives your life meaning. Interestingly, having a sense of purpose tends to encourage behaviors that support better health.

What gives you a sense of purpose?

- Family and close relationships
- Community involvement
- Helping others
- Learning new things
- Hobbies and creative pursuits
- Or maybe a combination of these

Purpose has a ripple effect. It influences your other wellness pillars like diet, exercise, and social connection. People with a strong sense of purpose are more likely to eat well, sleep better, stay active, and maintain strong relationships. Purpose also reduces stress, which in turn lowers inflammation, one of the biggest drivers of aging and chronic disease.

So, how do you find your purpose?

One beautiful tool is Ikigai, a Japanese concept meaning "a reason for being." It's your reason to wake up each day feeling alive and inspired. Ikigai is found at the intersection of four things:

- What you love—your passion
- What you are good at—your talents and strengths
- What the world needs—how you contribute
- What you can be paid for—your vocation or profession

When you align all four, you tap into something powerful. This place of inspiration doesn't just elevate your mental or emotional state; it positively impacts your biology. A life driven by purpose is a life that resists aging, builds resilience, and sustains vitality.

Let's Talk About Stress

Stress isn't just a feeling; it's a major factor in your long-term health. Chronic stress is directly linked to a wide range of health challenges, including:

- Anxiety disorders
- Depression
- Cardiovascular disease
- Autoimmune conditions
- Alzheimer's disease
- Certain types of cancer
- Systemic inflammation
- And many other age-related illnesses

So what can we do about it?

Here's the good news: the tools are simple. The challenge? Many people view them as a "waste of time," "unproductive," or say things like, "I'm just not good at it."

We're talking about breath work, meditation, and visualization. Now, before your eyes roll and you think "Here we go again," I want to ask you an honest question:

What is stress costing you?

- Your physical health?
- Your mental clarity?

- Your relationships?
- Your ability to succeed?
- Your capacity to make calm, confident decisions?

Take a moment to reflect on where your life is today because of stress, and where it could be if your stress levels were lower.

Let's do a little bit of a deeper dive!

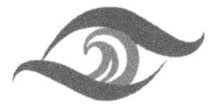

Rewire, Recharge, Reimagine

Train the Mind, Heal the Body, Shift the Biology

Meditation has been shown in countless studies to reduce:
- Inflammatory markers
- Anxiety and mild to moderate depression
- Pain
- Sleep disturbances

And to improve:
- Digestion
- Mood
- Focus
- Emotional balance

Meditation has been studied extensively in recent years, and the science is finally catching up with what ancient traditions have known for centuries. The core message across most meditation books is that regular meditation reshapes the brain and body in measurable ways.

Research shows that consistent practice can reduce stress, lower inflammation, improve emotional regulation, and even alter brain structure, increasing gray matter in areas responsible for memory, empathy, and self-awareness.

Meditation also reduces activity in the brain's default mode network (DMN), which is associated with mind-wandering and rumination. Different styles of meditation, such as mindfulness, loving-kindness, or focused attention, each offer unique benefits, but all help train the mind to become more present, less reactive, and more attuned to the moment.

Ultimately, meditation isn't about escaping your life; it's about learning to be fully alive within it. Here are a few different styles of meditation and their unique benefits:

1. **Mindfulness Meditation**—Originating from Buddhist traditions, this involves observing thoughts, emotions, and sensations without judgment. It helps reduce stress, improve focus, and enhance emotional regulation.

2. **Loving-Kindness Meditation (Metta)**—This style focuses on cultivating compassion and sending goodwill to yourself and others. It's been shown to increase positive emotions, empathy, and emotional resilience.

3. **Transcendental Meditation**—A mantra-based technique practiced twice daily for 20 minutes. It promotes deep relaxation, reduces anxiety, and improves heart health and overall cognitive function.

4. **Body Scan Meditation**—Involves slowly scanning the body for tension and releasing it. This practice helps with pain management, stress relief, and connecting more deeply with your physical body.

5. **Breath Awareness Meditation**—Focuses solely on the breath. It helps anchor the mind, improve concentration, and regulate the nervous system, making it a great entry point for beginners.
6. **Walking Meditation**—Combines movement with mindfulness by bringing awareness to each step. It enhances presence, improves circulation, and is especially useful for those who struggle with sitting still.
7. **Guided Visualization**—Uses imagery led by a teacher or recording to bring about relaxation or manifest goals. It can reduce anxiety, enhance creativity, and help with goal-setting or healing.

Each of these styles can be adapted to suit personal needs and goals, whether it's calming the mind, boosting compassion, or supporting physical and emotional healing.

So then the question becomes: how much and how often should you meditate to get the benefits? Well, that depends on your goals, lifestyle, and experience level, but here are general guidelines:

- For beginners: Start with 5–10 minutes a day, ideally at the same time each day (morning or evening works well). Consistency matters more than duration in the beginning. Even a measly one minute of just facing the sun and smiling will be incredibly effective to start.
- For stress relief and mental clarity: Aim for 10–20 minutes daily. This amount is supported by research showing improvements in mood, focus, and emotional regulation.

- For deeper transformation, like reducing anxiety, improving sleep, or cultivating mindfulness: Try 20–30 minutes once or twice a day. Many formal programs, like Transcendental Meditation, recommend two 20-minute sessions daily.

- For maintenance: Even five minutes of mindful breathing or awareness practice during a lunch break or before bed can help anchor your nervous system and provide benefits.

Ultimately, the best meditation routine is the one you can stick to consistently. It's better to meditate a little each day than to aim for perfection and skip days, which turn into weeks, which turn into months, which turn into ... well, you get the point!

The Free Medicine You've Been Ignoring

Breathwork (especially when done regularly) can:

- Improve mood and memory
- Lower blood pressure
- Boost alertness and creativity
- Enhance sleep
- Deepen relaxation
- Raise heart rate variability (a marker of resilience)
- Reduce stress from both physical and emotional sources

In *Breath: The New Science of a Lost Art,* James Nestor reveals how something as simple and automatic as breathing has been forgotten and how this neglect is affecting our health. He explores the science and history of breathing. Did you even think there would be a history to breathing? Well, there is, and it's fascinating!

It starts way, way back in the day, but one of the factors that started the changes to our facial structures is the creation of fire. Once we could use fire to cook food, we didn't have to chew as hard for as long or as much. Cooked food is softer, more nutrient-dense, and easier to chew and digest.

That change in diet led to big evolutionary shifts; our jaw lines and teeth became smaller, which then reduced our nasal and airway passages. This, in turn, caused most modern humans to develop poor habits like mouth breathing, which can lead to sleep disorders, high blood pressure, fatigue, and anxiety. This is all just because of this little thing that we use every day for multiple reasons . . . fire!

Did you know that after just 10 days of proper nose breathing and holding your tongue at the roof of your mouth, you can start changing your whole facial structure, *in just 10 days*. . . I mean, wow! Nasal breathing filters air, regulates temperature, and improves oxygen delivery throughout the body.

Ancient breathing practices and modern research indicate the benefits of slower, deeper, and more intentional breathing. Techniques such as Buteyko, box breathing, and the Wim Hof method are incredibly powerful tools that will improve your resilience, immunity, and mental clarity.

How we breathe is just as important as what we eat or how we move. Did you know that there is a magic anti-anxiety point on the roof of your mouth, right behind your top teeth? It's true! Place the tip of your tongue at that point and then lie the rest of your tongue across your palate, place your lips together, and breathe slowly into your belly. You should start to feel your anxiety melt away almost instantaneously. Here are a few more of my favorite breathing techniques.

Nasal Breathing

How: Simply close your mouth and breathe in and out through your nose.

Why: This is the default healthy breathing method. It filters, warms, and humidifies air, increases nitric oxide (which improves circulation), and slows down the breath for better oxygen delivery.

Use for: Everyday health, better sleep, less anxiety, improved endurance.

Box Breathing (aka Tactical Breathing)

How: Inhale for 4 seconds → hold for 4 seconds → exhale for 4 seconds → hold for 4 seconds.

Why: Helps regulate the nervous system by increasing parasympathetic (calming) tone.

Use for: Stress relief, anxiety, mental focus. Popular with Navy SEALs and first responders.

Wim Hof Breathing

How: Take 30 deep, fast breaths (in through the nose, out through the mouth) → hold breath after the last exhale → inhale and hold again for 15 seconds. Repeat for three rounds.

Why: This hyper-oxygenates the body and activates adrenaline and immune responses.

Use for: Building resilience, reducing inflammation, improving cold tolerance.

4-7-8 Breathing

How: Inhale for 4 seconds → hold for 7 seconds → exhale slowly for 8 seconds.

Why: Helps lower heart rate, calm the mind, and prepare the body for sleep.

Use for: Falling asleep faster, reducing stress, or emotional reactivity.

Buteyko Breathing

How: Breathe lightly through your nose with very shallow inhales and exhales, often followed by breath holds.

Why: Helps retrain the body to tolerate more carbon dioxide, which improves oxygen delivery and reduces overbreathing.

Use for: Asthma, anxiety, panic attacks, and chronic hyperventilation.

Diaphragmatic (Belly) Breathing

How: Place a hand on your belly. As you inhale, allow your belly to expand. Exhale slowly, and let the belly fall.

Why: Activates the vagus nerve, reduces cortisol, and oxygenates the lower lungs.

Use for: Managing stress, improving digestion, calming the body during rest or yoga.

Alternate Nostril Breathing (Nadi Shodhana)

How: Close the right nostril and inhale through the left → close the left, exhale through the right → inhale right, exhale left. Repeat.

Why: Balances the left and right brain hemispheres and reduces stress.

Use for: Mental clarity, emotional balance, preparing for meditation or sleep.

You can also try mouth taping, a simple yet powerful practice that encourages nasal breathing during sleep by gently sealing the lips with a piece of breathable tape. The idea behind it is rooted in both ancient breathing techniques and modern science: breathing through your nose rather than your mouth.

I am sure that very few of you have heard of Falim, am I right!? It is a Turkish brand of chewing gum that's often recommended by dentists, myofunctional therapists, and breathing experts, not because it tastes amazing (it's flavorless or mildly so), but because of how tough it is to chew.

Unlike regular gum, Falim is sugar-free, long-lasting, and significantly firmer, which makes it excellent for strengthening the jaw muscles and improving oral posture.

Chewing tough gum like Falim can help support:

- Proper tongue placement, which is essential for nasal breathing.
- Facial development in children and teens (a firmer jawline, better bite alignment).

- Mouth muscle tone, which can help reduce snoring and sleep apnea symptoms.
- Myofunctional therapy exercises, especially for people working on breathing or speech patterns.

Because Falim is so firm, it's best to ease into it—start with a few minutes a day and gradually increase. It's a simple, affordable tool to help retrain the way you use your mouth and support better breathing and sleep.

The Science of Seeing It Before You Become It

Visualization is our first and one of our most powerful tools for creating change from the inside out. Interestingly, studies have found that our ability to imagine, especially as we become older adults, tends to decline. This decline is linked to cognitive issues and reduced memory.

Visualization is more than just "thinking positive." It's about mentally living your desired outcome as if it's already happened. See it. Feel it. Walk through the scenario. But most importantly:

- Feel the emotions of already having it.
- Show gratitude as if it has already happened.

That emotional engagement is where the magic happens. We'll dive deeper into these practices in a later chapter. But for now, start simple.

Take a few minutes each day to visualize your healthiest, most vibrant self.

What are you doing?

Where are you?

Who are you with?

What are you accomplishing?

How does that feel?

Because the life you imagine is often the first step toward the life you create.

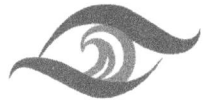

The Mirror Lies, Your Cells Don't

Biological Age Self Assessment (BASA)

Welcome to your next two assessments. Did you know that we have a word that describes inflammation in old age? Inflammaging is the term used to describe the chronic, low-grade inflammation that naturally develops as we age.

Unlike the short bursts of inflammation that help the body heal from injury or fight infection, inflammaging is persistent and subtle, silently damaging cells and tissues over time. This ongoing inflammatory state is now understood to be a major contributor to many age-related diseases, including heart disease, type 2 diabetes, Alzheimer's, and even cancer.

Factors that fuel inflammaging are poor diet, chronic stress, lack of sleep, toxin exposure, sedentary lifestyle, and gut dysbiosis. The good news is that lifestyle changes, like eating anti-inflammatory foods, supporting your gut health, getting restorative sleep, managing stress, and staying physically active, can dramatically reduce this harmful inflammation and slow the aging process at the cellular level. And guess what? This is the whole theme of this book . . . you're welcome!

Let's check in and see what your biological age is. How young are you really on the inside? This is your opportunity to track real progress and see how your choices are influencing your health and longevity. You can repeat this assessment every six months to monitor improvements.

Ready to start your BASA and see how youthful you truly are?

Section 1: Food & Nutrition

1. Veggie intake (1 serving = ~½ cup cooked or 1 cup raw):
   - ☐ None (+3)
   - ☐ 1–3 per day (+2)
   - ☐ 4–6 per day (-2)
   - ☐ 7+ per day (-3)

2. Nutrient-dense staples (nuts, seeds, eggs, fatty fish, or organ meats):
   - ☐ Rarely / once a month (+2)
   - ☐ Once per week (0)
   - ☐ 2–3 times per week (-2)
   - ☐ Almost daily (-3)

3. Fermented or prebiotic-rich foods (kimchi, sauerkraut, garlic, onion, kombucha, legumes):
   - ☐ Rarely (+2)
   - ☐ Once a week (0)
   - ☐ 2–3 times per week (-1)
   - ☐ Daily (-2)

4. Healing herbs & teas (turmeric, rosemary, garlic, green tea, matcha, curcumin/EGCG):
   - ☐ Rarely (+2)
   - ☐ 2–3 times per week (0)
   - ☐ Almost daily (-2)

5. Water intake per day:
   - ☐ 0 (+2)
   - ☐ 1–3 glasses (+1)
   - ☐ 4–7 glasses (0)
   - ☐ 8+ glasses (-1)

6. Longest daily fasting window (time between meals):
   - ☐ 9 hours or less (+1)
   - ☐ 10–12 hours (0)
   - ☐ 12+ hours (-1)

7. Mindful eating (away from screens, chew slowly, pause to breathe, savor food):
   - ☐ Never (+2)
   - ☐ Rarely (+1)
   - ☐ Sometimes (0)
   - ☐ Often (-1)

8. Alcohol per week (4 oz. wine or equivalent):
   - ☐ More than 21 drinks (+3)
   - ☐ 14–21 drinks (+2)
   - ☐ 5–14 drinks (+1)
   - ☐ Less than 5 drinks (-1)

9. Fried, broiled, or charred foods:
   - ☐ Almost daily (+2)
   - ☐ 2–3 times per week (+1)
   - ☐ Once per week (0)
   - ☐ Once per month or less (-1)

10. Refined sugar & flour (soda, pastries, packaged snacks, fast food):
    - ☐ Almost daily (+2)
    - ☐ 2–3 times per week (+1)
    - ☐ Once per week (0)
    - ☐ Once per month or less (-1)

Section 2: Lifestyle & Movement

1. Play (fun, unstructured activity—games, sports, laughter, hobbies):
   - ☐ Never (+2)
   - ☐ Once a month (0)
   - ☐ 1–2 times per week (-2)
   - ☐ 3+ times per week (-3)

2. Cardio (sweaty, hard-to-talk pace):
   - ☐ Never (+2)
   - ☐ Once a month (0)
   - ☐ 1–2 times per week (-2)
   - ☐ 3+ times per week (-3)

3. Strength training (weights, pushups, resistance bands):
   - ☐ Once a month (+1)
   - ☐ 1–2 times per week (-1)
   - ☐ 3+ times per week (-2)

4. Daily sitting time:
   - ☐ 8+ hours (+2)
   - ☐ 5–8 hours (+1)
   - ☐ Less than 5 hours (0)

5. Hours of sleep per night:
   - ☐ 0–4 (+2)
   - ☐ 5–6 (+1)
   - ☐ 7–9 (-2)
   - ☐ 10+ (+1)

6. Sleep quality:
   - ☐ Poor (+2)
   - ☐ Fair (+1)
   - ☐ Good (-1)

7. Toxin exposure (plastics, pollution, chemicals, cleaning products, dental mercury):
   - ☐ Very high (+3)
   - ☐ High (+2)
   - ☐ Moderate (+1)
   - ☐ Low (0)

8. Smoking or secondhand smoke:
   - ☐ 1 pack/day (+3)
   - ☐ Half pack/day (+2)
   - ☐ 1–5 cigarettes/day (+1)
   - ☐ None (0)

9. Former smoker (quit):
   - ☐ <1 year ago (+3)
   - ☐ 1–5 years ago (+2)
   - ☐ 6–10 years ago (+1)
   - ☐ 10+ years ago (0)

10. Time in nature (yard, park, hike, beach, etc.):
    - ☐ Rarely (+2)
    - ☐ 1–3x/month (0)
    - ☐ 1–3x/week (-1)
    - ☐ Daily (-2)

Section 3: Mental & Emotional Wellness

1. Stress frequency:
   - ☐ Daily (+2)
   - ☐ Weekly (+1)
   - ☐ Monthly (-1)
   - ☐ Rarely (-2)

2. Stress coping strategies:
   - ☐ Meditation, breathwork, journaling, talking (-2)
   - ☐ Exercise (-1)

- ☐ Comfort food (+1)
- ☐ Smoking/drinking (+2)
- ☐ Medications (tranquilizers, antidepressants) (+3)

3. Overall happiness:
   - ☐ Mostly unhappy (+2)
   - ☐ Sometimes unhappy (+1)
   - ☐ Generally happy (-1)
   - ☐ Mostly happy (-2)

4. Number of strong, reliable relationships:
   - ☐ None (+2)
   - ☐ Few (+1)
   - ☐ Some (-1)
   - ☐ Many (-2)

5. Work satisfaction:
   - ☐ Not at all (+2)
   - ☐ Somewhat (+1)
   - ☐ Mostly (-1)
   - ☐ Love it (-2)

6. Community involvement:
   - ☐ Very active (-2)
   - ☐ Somewhat (-1)
   - ☐ Not much (+1)
   - ☐ Not at all (+2)

7. Creativity (art, music, writing, DIY projects, crafts, etc.):
   - ☐ Daily (-2)

☐ Weekly (-1)
☐ Rarely/never (+1)

8. Learning new skills (languages, instruments, new field of study):
   ☐ Yes (-3)
   ☐ No (0)

9. Sense of purpose in life:
   ☐ Always (-2)
   ☐ Sometimes (-1)
   ☐ Rarely (+1)
   ☐ Never (+2)

10. Spiritual practice (prayer, meditation, stillness, gratitude):
    ☐ Daily (-2)
    ☐ Weekly (-1)
    ☐ Rarely (0)

Section 4: Body Measurements

1. Waist circumference
   ☐ Male >40" / Female >35" (+2)
   ☐ Male 37–39" / Female 33–34" (+1)
   ☐ Male 32–36" / Female 28–32" (0)
   ☐ Male <32" / Female <28" (-1)

2. BMI (check at nhlbi.nih.gov/calculate-your-bmi)
   ☐ 35+ (+3)
   ☐ 31–34 (+2)

☐ 20–30 (0)
☐ <20 (+1)

3. Blood pressure (diastolic = bottom number):
   ☐ 90+ (+2)
   ☐ 80–89 (+1)
   ☐ 60–79 (-1)

Calculating Your Bio-Age Shift

1. Total up the number, positive and negative.
2. Divide by 10 (just add a decimal point. For example, if your total is -12, your score is -1.2).
3. Subtract this number from (or add it to) your chronological age to find out your bio age. If you can get to seven years younger biologically compared to your chronological age, you decrease your risk of disease by 50%. The younger your biological age, the less risk of disease you have.

Example: Age 45 with score of -15 → -1.5 → Bio age = 43.5.

TruDiagnostic's TruAge Test

If you want the most accurate insight into your biological age, I recommend starting with the in-depth TruAge test by TruDiagnostic: www.trudiagnostic.com/

Here's how to get the most from your testing:

1. Start with the comprehensive TruAge test before making any major changes; this gives you a solid baseline.

2. At six months, follow up with the DunedinPACE test to see how your rate of aging is responding to your lifestyle, diet, and exercise changes.
3. At 12 months, do the full TruAge test again to track long-term shifts in your biological age.

Remember, chronological age is just a number. Your biological age reflects the real story of your body's resilience, regeneration, and overall health.

Medical Screening Symptoms Questionnaire

Welcome to the MSQ—Medical Symptoms Questionnaire. This is one of the most widely used tools by Functional Medicine practitioners around the world to track your progress and response to treatment.[4]

Here's how it works:

- Rate each of the symptoms listed based on your experience over the past seven days.
- At the end of each section, add up your score.
- Calculate your grand total score.

The goal is to see that grand total score go down over time, showing that your body is healing, rebalancing, and responding to all the good things you're doing for it.

You can complete this questionnaire monthly to check in with yourself, stay motivated, and celebrate your wins along your health journey!

---

[4] The Institute for Functional Medicine, accessed August 24, 2025, https://www.ifm.org/articles/the-ifm-toolkit.

Let's get started. Your body is always talking to you, and this is one way to listen.

Rate each of the following symptoms based on your typical health profile for the past seven days.

Point Scale:
0 (Never or almost never have the symptom)
3 (Frequently have it, effect is not severe)
1 (Occasionally have it, effect is not severe)
4 (Frequently have it, effect is severe)
2 (Occasionally have it, effect is severe)

HEAD
☐ Headaches
☐ Faintness
☐ Dizziness
☐ Insomnia

TOTAL _____

EYES
☐ Watery or itchy eyes
☐ Swollen, reddened, or sticky eyelids
☐ Bags or dark circles under the eyes
☐ Blurred or tunnel vision

TOTAL _____

EARS
- ☐ Itchy ears
- ☐ Earache, ear infections
- ☐ Draining from the ear
- ☐ Ringing in the ears, hearing loss

TOTAL _____

NOSE
- ☐ Stuffy nose
- ☐ Sinus problems
- ☐ Hay Fever
- ☐ Sneezing attacks
- ☐ Excessive mucus formation

TOTAL _____

MOUTH/THROAT
- ☐ Chronic cough
- ☐ Gagging, frequent need to clear throat
- ☐ Sore throat, hoarseness, loss of voice
- ☐ Swollen or discolored tongue, gums, lips
- ☐ Canker sores

TOTAL _____

SKIN
- ☐ Acne
- ☐ Hives, rashes, dry skin
- ☐ Hair loss

- ☐ Flushing, hot flashes
- ☐ Excessive sweating

TOTAL _____

HEART

- ☐ Irregular or skipped heartbeat
- ☐ Rapid or pounding heartbeat
- ☐ Chest pain

TOTAL _____

LUNGS

- ☐ Chest congestion
- ☐ Asthma, bronchitis
- ☐ Shortness of breath
- ☐ Difficulty breathing

TOTAL _____

DIGESTIVE TRACT

- ☐ Nausea, vomiting
- ☐ Diarrhea
- ☐ Constipation
- ☐ Bloated feeling
- ☐ Belching, passing gas
- ☐ Heartburn
- ☐ Intestinal/stomach pain

TOTAL _____

JOINT/MUSCLE
- ☐ Pain or aches in joints
- ☐ Arthritis
- ☐ Stiffness or limitation of movement
- ☐ Pain or aches in muscles
- ☐ Feeling of weakness or tiredness

TOTAL _____

WEIGHT
- ☐ Binge eating/drinking
- ☐ Craving certain foods
- ☐ Excessive weight
- ☐ Compulsive eating
- ☐ Water retention
- ☐ Underweight

TOTAL _____

ENERGY/ACTIVITY
- ☐ Fatigue, sluggishness
- ☐ Apathy, lethargy
- ☐ Hyperactivity
- ☐ Restlessness

TOTAL _____

MIND
- ☐ Poor memory
- ☐ Confusion, poor comprehension

☐ Poor concentration
☐ Difficulty making decisions
☐ Stuttering or stammering
☐ Slurred speech
☐ Learning disabilities

TOTAL _____

EMOTIONS
☐ Mood swings
☐ Anxiety, fear, nervousness
☐ Anger, irritability, aggressiveness
☐ Depression

TOTAL _____

OTHER
☐ Frequent illness
☐ Frequent or urgent urination
☐ Genital itch or discharge

TOTAL _____

GRAND TOTAL _____

Interpreting your results:

Less than 10: Aging at an optimal rate

10-50: Aging at a typical rate

50-100: Aging at a moderately accelerated rate

100+: Aging at a significantly accelerated rate

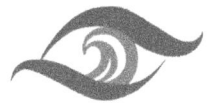

Beyond DNA: How Lifestyle Writes Your Genetic Story

The Tale of Two Mice

Let me tell you a little story about two mice. Same breed. Same genes. Same lab. But if you looked at them, you'd swear they came from two different planets.

One is lean, vibrant, and has the healthy brown color you'd expect. The other? Bright orange, overweight, and prone to all the big baddies: cancer, diabetes, and heart disease. But here's the plot twist: they are genetically identical.

Their difference came down to one thing: what their moms ate while pregnant.

Mama Mouse #1 ate regular old mouse chow. Her baby turned out orange and unhealthy.

Mama Mouse #2 got the same chow, but with a sprinkle of key nutrients: B9 (folate), B6, B12, choline, and a few others. Her baby? Lean, brown, and bursting with health.[5]

---

[5] Transposable elements: Targets for early nutritional effects on epigenetic gene regulation: Molecular and Cellular Biology: Vol 23, no 15, accessed August 24, 2025, https://www.tandfonline.com/doi/10.1128/MCB.23.15.5293-5300.2003?url_ver=Z39.88-2003&=&rfr_id=ori:rid:crossref.org&=&rfr_dat=cr_pub++0pubmed.

No magic. Just methylation, a natural process in your body that depends on nutrients to help control which of your genes are "on" and which stay "off."

Genetics vs. Epigenetics: The Game-Changer

Let's pause. What does this all mean? Your genetics are like the hand of cards you're dealt at birth: your eye color, hair type, and even your risk for certain diseases.

But your epigenetics? That's how you choose to play those cards. Epigenetics is like a dimmer switch for your genes, dialing them up or down. You can think of it as the "software" that tells your genes when to turn on or off. And the great news is that you're in control of the software through your:

- Diet
- Movement
- Stress management
- Sleep
- Environment
- Thoughts

It was thought that this was your destiny, and as we like to say to our kids, "You get what you get, and you don't get upset!"

WRONG!

Thank God our bodies are smarter than we are, because with just a little bit of guidance, our bodies can edit and reverse almost every moment of our lives. So even if you inherited genes that increase your risk for things like heart disease, diabetes, cancer, or depression, it doesn't mean you're doomed. It means you have the power to influence how those genes behave. So no, you are not doomed by your family history.

Here is the thing: your genes are writing your health story. Think of your genes as writers. Every single day, they're typing up the story of your health based on how you treat your body and mind.

If you eat nourishing foods, move your body, sleep well, and keep your stress in check, your genes write a beautiful chapter. You feel energized, your skin glows, your digestion works, and your mind is clear.

But if your lifestyle slips . . . say you're eating poorly, not moving, drowning in stress, and barely sleeping, your genes will still write, but the story might not be one you want to read.

Let's bring it to life:

- An older person who has used lots of steroid creams for years may have thin, fragile skin. Their genes are saying, "We're trying, but we don't have what we need to rebuild strong, healthy skin anymore."
- That person you know with glowing skin, thick hair, and boundless energy? Their genes are getting great instructions from their lifestyle.
- What about that guy that is strong and healthy, focuses on nutrient dense foods, has a great working gut, exercises multiple times per week, is a happy-go-lucky kind of guy, but then goes through a stressful time in life and starts only eating fast food, stops exercising, rarely gets

off the couch, sleeps poorly, and is really depressing to be around?

At this point, his genes are saying whoa, whoa, whoa, hold on a second, you are feeding me so much crap, I can't keep up with this! Until you change your ways again, I will write your story a little differently now. You're going to get a leaky gut, you will gain weight, your hair will start falling out, and your depression will get worse the longer you keep going with this diet and lifestyle, and . . . you're welcome!

Enter: SNPs (Single Nucleotide Polymorphisms)

Think of your genes like a giant instruction manual made up of billions of letters. Sometimes, a single letter gets swapped out, like a typo. That's an SNP (pronounced "snip").

There are over 10 million known SNPs in humans. Most of them are harmless typos, but some can change everything, from how you detox to how you absorb vitamins, even your personality and mood.

For example, the famous MTHFR SNP (yes, that's really what it's called) makes it harder for your body to use folate properly, a key player in methylation.

Here's the good news—even if you have SNPs, epigenetics can override them. Your body is not stuck with its instruction manual. You get to keep editing with every meal, every walk, every deep breath.

Wait, What's Methylation, You Ask?

Methylation is like a highlighter for your DNA. It adds tiny "tags" called methyl groups to certain genes, telling them to turn on or off. It doesn't change your genes; it changes how your body uses them.

And guess what fuels methylation? Your diet, your exercise plan, your lifestyle, your choices! That's why those extra nutrients during pregnancy made such a huge difference. They gave that baby mouse the best chance at a healthy, vibrant life.

Another way to look at it is that methylation is like your body's behind-the-scenes operations team. Every second, billions of methylation reactions are happening in every cell, flipping genetic switches on or off, producing energy, repairing DNA, detoxifying chemicals, balancing hormones, and even making you feel happy.

So, What Can Mess With Methylation?

- Poor nutrition (junk food, low B vitamins)
- Stress (hello, cortisol overload)
- Pollution and toxins
- Lack of exercise
- Certain SNPs (like MTHFR, COMT, BHMT)

When methylation goes off track, it can lead to:

- Brain fog and fatigue
- Anxiety or depression
- Hormonal imbalances

- Inflammation
- Faster aging
- Higher risk of chronic illness

But here's the thing: you can support methylation naturally. All you have to do is feed your genes right! Your body needs cofactors to methylate properly, mostly B vitamins and minerals. You will find them in:

- Leafy greens (hello, spinach and kale)
- Eggs (especially the yolk!)
- Beans and lentils
- Salmon and liver (if you're into that sort of thing)
- Beets, broccoli, and Brussels sprouts

Supplements can help if you have certain SNPs, but food first, always!

Methylation: The Aging Accelerator or Slower-Downer?

Methylation literally changes how fast you age. As you get older, your methylation tends to get—well, let's say—funky. Some bad genes (such as inflammation or cancer) get switched on. Some good ones (DNA repair, detox) get shut down. That's why we see aging-related diseases like:

- Alzheimer's
- Type 2 diabetes
- Heart disease
- Osteoporosis

- Cancer
- Autoimmunity
- Depression

Guess what? We now know that DNA methylation patterns can be measured to determine your "biological age," which may be way younger (or older) than your actual age . . . crazy, right?

Even if you are biologically older, it's okay, because epigenetics is reversible, even in older adults! Scientists used to think that once your genes were "set," that was it; you would just ride the wave and deal with whatever your body threw at you.

But we now know that epigenetics is like typing on a keyboard. Your DNA is the computer, and epigenetics is what you choose to write. You can delete, rewrite, and upgrade your story anytime. It's never too late to change the plot. Even cuddling, laughing, exercising, or meditating can positively influence your epigenome. Your lifestyle is your software update.

Powering It All Are the Mitochondria (The Unsung Heroes)

If methylation is the control room, then mitochondria are your power grid. These tiny powerhouses in your cells convert food into usable energy (ATP). The more energy you need, the more mitochondria your cells will have. We already mentioned it, but just to really get the point across:

- Heart cells have 5,000 mitochondria per cell.
- Liver 1,000–2,000
- Eggs have up to 600,000 mitochondria each!
- Sperm have a puny 20–75 (sorry, fellas).

And get this, your mitochondria have their own DNA, passed down only from your mom. So, yeah, female power goes all the way down to your cells. When your mitochondria become damaged (from aging, stress, or a poor diet), energy tanks. You may feel it as fatigue, brain fog, poor healing, and more. But when they're happy, you feel amazing, vibrant, sharp, and full of life.

So, let this sink in:

- 6 in 10 adults in the U.S. have a chronic disease
- 4 in 10 have two or more
- By age 80, the average person has five diseases and takes 5+ medications

We've been told that's "normal."

It's not!

It is common AND preventable.

You're not just aging. You're either aging gracefully or aging poorly, and that choice largely depends on your epigenetics, methylation, mitochondria, and yes, your daily choices.

Your Genes Are Listening

Every moment of every day, your genes are writing your story. We all get that at this point, right? Want clearer skin? Better moods? More energy? A longer healthspan? Then feed your body the tools it needs: love, nourishment, movement, rest, and purpose.

You're not stuck with the script you were given. You get to be the editor! You're not just a passenger in your genetic vehicle, you're the driver. So the real question is: What kind of story do you want your genes to write today?

Here is a quick introduction to a few of the genes you will be assessing yourself on to see which ones are "dirty" or switched off when they shouldn't be, or vice versa!

MTHFR

- Affects antioxidant production, brain chemistry, cell repair, detoxification, energy production, genetic expression, immune response, and inflammation
- Common signs are anxiety, brain fog, chemical sensitivity, depression, and irritability
- We need vitamins B2, B9, and B12; clean protein; magnesium to keep the genes healthy; lots of dark, leafy greens; and sleep is extremely important.

  Check your thyroid, and have the doctor check the full panel–there should be at least eight markers. Have them check the ranges against European ranges, not American. Additional supplements are L-5-MTHF or 6S-MTHF, but if you experience anxiety, irritability, a runny nose, joint pain, insomnia, or hives with these, please stop taking them.
- Avoid folic acid, industrial chemicals, heavy metals, alcohol, nitrous oxide, and sleep deprivation.

NOTE: Folic acid is the man-made form of vitamin B9 (often confused with folate). You find it in many supplements and fortified foods, but your body has to convert it into the active form (methylfolate) before it can use it.

Many people, especially those with an SNP on the MTHFR gene, aren't great at making that conversion. This can leave you with a buildup of unused folic acid, which may mess with how your body processes folate and even hide a vitamin B12 deficiency. You are better off getting folate naturally from leafy greens, beans, and avocados, or choose supplements with methylfolate so your body can put it to work right away.

COMT

- Slow COMT—Your body cannot clear estrogen, dopamine, epinephrine, and norepinephrine
- Fast COMT—Your body clears the above too quickly
- Common signs of slow COMT—high confidence; energy, enthusiasm; strong sexual function; estrogen issues—PMS, menstrual issues, fibroids, or higher risk of female cancers; irritability; pain intolerance; sleep difficulties; trouble relaxing; sensitive to caffeine and chocolate
- Common signs of fast COMT—calm, good-tempered, effective stress response, pain tolerance, difficulty completing tasks and focusing, forgetful, lack of confidence and optimism, low energy, menopause/perimenopause challenges
- You need vitamins B2, B9, and B12, clean protein, and magnesium to keep the genes healthy, with a particular importance on magnesium. You need to eat three healthy meals a day to help support your blood sugar levels, and eat only until you are 80% full. Stress management is very important; sauna, Epsom salt baths, and hot yoga are helpful.

Slow COMT

Optimizing your weight is very helpful for this dirty gene, along with eating beets, carrots, onions, artichokes, cruciferous vegetables, and bitter vegetables like dandelion root and radishes.

Be careful of the meds you are on; if you feel worse, contact your doctor and ask for a different medication if applicable. Anyone with this SNP may benefit from a lower-protein diet. Check your thyroid, and have the doctor check the *full* panel. There should be at least eight markers, and have them check the ranges against European ranges, not American! Additional supplementation includes adaptogens, taurine, SAMe, phosphatidyl serine, creatine, phosphatidylcholine, indole-3-carbinol, and DIM.

Fast COMT

Play music, dance, sing, participate in debates, go hiking, or play team sports; these types of activities tend to stimulate you and engage your brain.

Be aware of your addictive personality, meditate, do breathwork, or run! Medication and supplements that make slow COMT will make you much worse, so avoid the above list! Additional supplements include NADH, adrenal cortex, Tyrosine, and 5-HTP.

Avoid industrial chemicals, stress, depressing movies, the news, social media, and problematic friends.

NOTE: The goal isn't to make COMT faster or slower; it's to work with what you've got. A fast COMT may need more dopamine support to keep focus and motivation strong.

A slow COMT needs to focus on stress management and helping your body clear estrogen efficiently. Knowing your COMT type lets you play to your strengths and support your weak spots, so your brain, mood, and hormones stay in balance.

DAO

- You have a high reaction to histamine in your gut. You are more likely to develop sensitivities or allergic reactions to food. If the histamine is absorbed through your gut and increases at the cellular level, you are more likely to develop neurological disorders such as Parkinson's.

- Common signs are allergic reactions such as hives, runny nose, itchiness, food sensitivities, car sickness, seasickness, leaky gut, nausea, indigestion, pregnancy complications, and SIBO.

- If you score high on this gene, calcium and copper are the most important nutrients for you, as well as histamine blockers, vitamin C, and fish oils.

- Balance your meals so that your body's acid levels are low enough for the DAO enzyme to work. Sodium bicarbonate and potassium bicarbonate will serve you well if you have a diet high in acidic foods.

- Avoid stress as it will impact your stomach acid production, digestive enzymes, and bile. You are more prone to pathogenic bacteria entering your gut and causing issues, so clean your food correctly before eating.

MAOA

- Slow MAOA—Your body eliminates dopamine, norepinephrine, and serotonin more slowly
- Fast MAOA—Your body eliminates the above too quickly

- Common signs of slow MAOA—difficulty falling asleep, startles easily, headaches, irritability, mood swings, prolonged anxiety, rage and/or aggressive behavior, and trouble relaxing and powering down
- Common signs of fast MAOA—alcoholism and/or other addictions, ADHD, carb and sugar craving, depression, difficulty staying asleep, fatigue
- Vitamin B2 is the most important nutrient for cleaning this gene. You need to eat three protein-rich meals a day to help balance your neurotransmitters, balanced with healthy fats and some carbs. Limit sugar and processed foods, and do NOT overeat. Stress management is very important, as is good quality sleep.

Slow MAOA

You may have trouble with SSRIs, testosterone, certain thyroid medications, tryptophan, 5-HTP, melatonin, tyrosine, and inositol, so check the supplements that you are taking and adjust if needed.

Fast MAOA

Identify what is inflaming you and eliminate it; do not overtrain, and test yourself and your home for mold. Additional supplements include NADH, 5-HTP, inositol, melatonin, and liposomal curcumin.

Avoid stress, as this depletes your glutathione levels, and that makes you far more susceptible to holding onto heavy metals and other chemicals as they build up in your tissues, disrupt your detox pathways, and contribute to inflammation and cellular damage over time.

GST/GPX

- Your body is not able to attach glutathione (a master antioxidant) to xenobiotics (harmful environmental chemicals such as pesticides, herbicides, and heavy metals). They then build up in your tissues, disrupt your detox pathways, and contribute to inflammation and cellular damage over time.

- Common signs are hypersensitivity to chemicals (which includes symptoms such as congestion, runny nose, watery eyes, coughing, sneezing, fatigue, migraines, rashes, hives, digestive issues, anxiety, depression, and brain fog), increased inflammation, high blood pressure, and being overweight/obese.

- You will need B2, selenium, and cysteine to clean up this gene. Liposomal glutathione and detox powders are a must. Eat healthy fats and cut out processed foods, sugars, and add a moderate amount of protein (not too little and not too much). Eat a higher fiber diet to help detoxification. Dry brushing your skin and getting regular massages are amazing additions to your health routine.

- Avoid stress, and find and remove all possible infections in your body.

NOS3

- Your body isn't producing enough nitric oxide, which is vital for heart health. Without it, your blood vessels can't dilate properly, and your platelets can become overly sticky, both of which can increase the risk of blood clots.

- Common signs are angina, anxiety, cold hands and feet, depression, heart attack, erectile dysfunction, high blood pressure, migraines, mouth breathing, sinus congestion, and wounds that are slow to heal.
- You will need arginine, calcium, iron, vitamin B2, and glutathione to clean up this gene. Follow a low-inflammatory diet. Some sort of exercise, nose breathing, and breath work are very important. Sauna will benefit you as well. Additional supplements include ornithine, beet root powder, citrulline, PQQ, liposomal vitamin C, and liposomal glutathione.
- Avoid foods that contain folic acid. Avoid stress, as it will impact your neurotransmitters. You are also more prone to infections of all kinds. If possible, tape your mouth while you sleep, and teach yourself to nose breathe; it is one of the fastest ways to clean up this gene. Avoid chemical exposure.

PEMT

- Your body is unable to produce phosphatidylcholine; as a result, your cell membranes lose their integrity. They cannot absorb nutrients, your bile flow will not be smooth, and you have a higher risk of getting excess bacteria in your small intestine and a higher risk of developing fatty liver. It is also important for nerve function, muscle movement, and brain development. You may have low estrogen, so that needs to be supported either by hormone replacement therapy, supplementation, and/or diet. Check your cholesterol—low cholesterol will affect your estrogen production.

- Common signs are fatigue, fatty liver, gallbladder disorder, inflammation, muscle pain, malnourishment, pregnancy complications, SIBO, elevated triglycerides, and muscle weakness.
- You will need choline to clean up this gene. Phosphatidylcholine and creatine are also great additions. If you have a leaky gut, you will need to heal it to reduce the pathogenic bacteria that can cause all sorts of problems in your metabolism, inflammation levels, and detox pathways, ultimately helping to lower the toxic load on your body and prevent further genetic expression issues.
- Physical and emotional stress burn through choline, so stress management is key.

BHMT

- Your body produces too much homocysteine, and too much can damage blood vessels and increase your risk for heart disease, stroke, and cognitive decline. It also creates methionine, which is an essential amino acid used to make SAMe (S-adenosylmethionine), your body's main methyl donor, as well as proteins, neurotransmitters, and antioxidants.
- Common signs are general inflammation, anxiety and depression, fatigue, fullness after eating fats, nausea after eating fats, and insomnia.
- You will need choline, betaine, zinc, B6, B12, and folate to clean up this gene. Make sure your detox pathways are working (regular bowel movements, appropriate sweating, and regular urination). Practice stress management and get good quality sleep. Check your gut and

hormone health because you want to avoid high estrogen levels.
- Avoid physical and emotional stress, industrial chemicals, and heavy metals.

CBS

- Your body has a hard time detoxing and handles certain nutrients and toxins, particularly sulfur, ammonia, and homocysteine, poorly. You also have a hard time producing glutathione, your body's master antioxidant.
- Common signs are headaches or migraines, muscle pain, fatigue, trouble detoxing (especially sulfur-based supplements or meds), sensitivity to sulfur-rich foods, digestive issues, brain fog, anxiety, irritability, and ADD.
- You will need magnesium, B12, folate, zinc, molybdenum, liposomal glutathione, NAC, and then L-ornithine, charcoal, and B6 to help with detox pathways.
- Avoid physical and emotional stress, industrial chemicals, heavy metals, and a diet rich in sulfur.

MTR

- If you have low B12, this gene will work more slowly, which will in turn affect your hormones, neurotransmitters, and detox pathways.
- Common signs are headaches or migraines, insomnia, brain fog, fatigue, depression and anxiety, tingling in the arms or legs, and getting sick easily.
- You will need magnesium, B12, folate (5-MTHF), zinc, trimethylglycine or betaine, and choline.

- Avoid physical and emotional stress, B12 forms such as cyanocobalamin, and start with a low dose of B vitamins and slowly build up.

SHMT

- Your body produces less folate, which impairs DNA synthesis and throws your neurotransmitters out of balance.
- Common signs are insomnia, brain fog, fatigue, depression and anxiety, hormonal imbalances, slow wound healing, getting stressed out easily, and fertility issues.
- You will need 5-MTHF, B6 (P5P form), glycine and serine, magnesium, zinc, B12 (methylcobalamin), choline, and liposomal glutathione.
- Avoid physical and emotional stress, and high-folic-acid foods.

Is One of Your Genes Acting Up?

We all have genes that do important jobs like clearing toxins, managing stress, producing energy, and balancing mood. But when those genes get "dirty" from a poor diet, chronic stress, lack of sleep, or environmental overload, they don't work as well. A "dirty" gene doesn't mean something's broken. It just means that your body needs a little extra support.

This quick assessment will help you spot signs that certain genes like MTHFR, COMT, MAOA, DAO, GST, PEMT, and a few others may be under strain. Once you know where your weak spots are, you can clean them up with the right foods, lifestyle upgrades, and targeted support. So, let's find out which of your genes could use a little spring cleaning.

Check the box if the condition has occurred frequently within the last 60 days or is generally true: Award one point per question.

MTHFR & Methylation Self Check

Tick off the statements that sound like you. This isn't about labels or diagnoses; it's about noticing patterns that may give you clues into how your body handles energy, mood, and detox.

Mood & Mind

- ☐ I've experienced headaches that come and go without a clear reason.
- ☐ My mood sometimes swings between irritability and feeling low.
- ☐ I notice I can concentrate well—unless my emotions (anger, sadness, stress) get in the way.
- ☐ I've had periods of depression, anxiety, or irritability that seem tied to stress or lifestyle.

Energy & Recovery

- ☐ I often feel drained, sluggish, or "toxic," even without being sick.
- ☐ After a workout, I sometimes get flushed, short of breath, or even wheezy.
- ☐ It can take me a while to wind down and feel calm after getting upset.
- ☐ Falling asleep isn't always easy. I sometimes feel wired at night.

Nutrition & Lifestyle

- ☐ I don't eat leafy green vegetables every day.
- ☐ I've taken supplements or eaten foods enriched with folic acid (not folate from greens).
- ☐ Alcohol doesn't sit well with me—I feel it faster or worse than others.
- ☐ Nitrous oxide (laughing gas) at the dentist made me feel unusually bad.

Body Signals

- ☐ My hands and feet often feel cold.
- ☐ I sweat easily and heavily during exercise.

DAO & Histamine Sensitivity Self-Check

Place a check mark by each statement that resonates with you. DAO (diamine oxidase) is the enzyme your body uses to break down histamine from food. If your DAO is sluggish, histamine can build up, triggering all sorts of frustrating symptoms.

Food & Drink Reactions

- ☐ I notice symptoms (irritability, sweating, runny nose, nosebleeds, or headaches) after eating leftovers, fish, citrus, or fermented foods.
- ☐ Red wine, beer, or alcohol makes me feel worse than I should.
- ☐ I don't tolerate yogurt, kefir, cheese, chocolate, or fermented foods very well.
- ☐ I can't tolerate certain probiotics.

Gut & Immune Clues

- ☐ I've been told I have leaky gut, SIBO, Crohn's disease, or ulcerative colitis.
- ☐ I have many food allergies or intolerances.
- ☐ I generally feel better a few hours *after* eating than I do right after a meal.
- ☐ I felt more resilient during pregnancy and could eat more foods than usual.

Skin, Lungs & Mood

- ☐ I often feel itchy, flushed, or overheated after meals.
- ☐ If I scratch my skin, it leaves red streaks.
- ☐ I've experienced hives, eczema, psoriasis, or unexplained rashes.
- ☐ I sometimes get asthma or exercise-induced asthma.
- ☐ I deal with migraines or headaches regularly.
- ☐ I get random, moving joint pain that comes and goes.
- ☐ I sometimes hear ringing in my ears, especially after meals.
- ☐ I have a runny or congested nose often, or occasional nosebleeds.
- ☐ I struggle to fall asleep if I've eaten or had alcohol too close to bedtime.

COMT "Slow" Self-Check

Check the statements that sound familiar. Your COMT gene helps your body break down stress chemicals and certain hormones. If COMT runs on the "slower" side, you may process adrenaline, estrogen, and dopamine at a snail's pace, leading to mood swings, tension, and sleep struggles.

Sleep & Mood

- ☐ I have a hard time falling asleep, sometimes lying awake for hours replaying the day.
- ☐ I've struggled with sleep issues since childhood. (I could describe my ceiling in detail!)
- ☐ I get headaches, especially during times of stress or hormone shifts.
- ☐ I often feel anxious, irritable, or impatient.
- ☐ Once I get upset, it takes me a while to calm down.
- ☐ Caffeine wakes me up, but too much makes me edgy or snappy.

Hormones & PMS

- ☐ PMS has been (or used to be) a big issue for me.
- ☐ My doctor once suggested birth control pills for acne, heavy bleeding, or PMS.
- ☐ I have, or have had, uterine fibroids.
- ☐ I notice that hormone fluctuations really affect my mood, energy, or focus.

Food & Focus

- ☐ High-protein diets (like Paleo or GAPS) sometimes leave me more irritable.
- ☐ I'm sensitive to pain and don't handle discomfort well.
- ☐ I can focus and study for long hours—but at the cost of becoming wound up or tense.

Personality & Tendencies

- ☐ I'm generally happy and enthusiastic, but I get irritated easily.
- ☐ I tend to be cautious rather than a risk-taker.
- ☐ I know I'm not the most patient person in the room.

COMT "Fast" Self-Check

Check any statements that sound like you. COMT is the gene that helps clear stress chemicals, estrogen, and dopamine. If you've got a "fast" COMT, your system may be clearing these brain chemicals too quickly—leading to focus struggles, low motivation, and the need for extra stimulation to feel balanced.

Focus & Motivation

- ☐ I often struggle with paying attention or staying focused.
- ☐ Getting going in the morning is tough for me—I feel sluggish until I get a boost.
- ☐ I lack motivation or feel low energy about starting things.
- ☐ Caffeine helps me concentrate and get into gear.

Mood & Behavior

- ☐ I'm prone to dips in mood or feelings of depression.
- ☐ I sometimes feel better after eating carbs or sweets—but the slump comes back fast.
- ☐ I crave high-fat, high-sugar comfort foods, and while they help briefly, the effect doesn't last.
- ☐ Most of the time, I'm calm under stress, but I can also feel kind of flat emotionally.

Personality & Habits

- ☐ I'm a natural risk-taker and love the adrenaline rush of stunts or challenges.
- ☐ I've got a "class clown" side—I love making people laugh and being the center of attention.
- ☐ I tend to fidget, move constantly, or need something to do with my hands.
- ☐ I've even pinched myself hard just to feel something stimulating.
- ☐ I don't have a high interest in sex compared to others.

Addiction & Stimulation

- ☐ I find myself easily hooked on activities or substances—like gaming, shopping, smoking, alcohol, social media, or gambling.
- ☐ I get a rush from these behaviors, but it doesn't take long before I need the next "hit."

Sleep

- ☐ When it's bedtime, I usually crash right away—my head hits the pillow and I'm out.

MAOA "Slow" Self-Check

The MAOA gene helps your body clear out serotonin, dopamine, and norepinephrine, the brain chemicals that regulate mood, focus, and stress. If you have the "slow" type, these brain messengers may hang around too long, leading to anxiety, irritability, and difficulty calming down. Tick the boxes that sound like you.

Stress & Mood

- ☐ I get stressed, panicked, or anxious more easily than others.
- ☐ When I do get upset, it takes me a while to calm down.
- ☐ I can be more aggressive or irritable under pressure.
- ☐ Caffeine tends to make me edgy or more irritable.
- ☐ SSRIs (prescribed for depression) made me feel more agitated instead of calmer.
- ☐ Lithium tends to help stabilize my mood.
- ☐ Supplements like 5-HTP or inositol overstimulate me or make me feel worse.

Focus & Personality

- ☐ Once I lock into something, I can focus for long stretches.
- ☐ I tend to carry myself with confidence.
- ☐ I'm less drawn to carbs compared to others, and feel more stable when I don't eat many.

Food & Drink

- ☐ I enjoy foods like cheese, wine, and chocolate—but I often feel "off," irritable, or moody after consuming them.
- ☐ Alcohol can bring out the angry side of me instead of making me relaxed.

Sleep

- ☐ Falling asleep can be difficult, but once I'm out, I usually sleep through the night.

MAOA "Fast" Self-Check

The MAOA gene helps break down serotonin, dopamine, and norepinephrine, your "feel-good" brain messengers. If your MAOA enzyme is fast, it clears them out too quickly, which can leave you running low. The result? Low mood, restless sleep, carb cravings, and trouble focusing.

Check off the statements that feel familiar.

Sleep Patterns

- ☐ I fall asleep quickly, but often wake up earlier than I'd like.
- ☐ I sometimes wake during the night and need a snack to fall back asleep.
- ☐ Melatonin works well for me when I need help with sleep.

Mood & Emotions

- ☐ I'm prone to depression or a lack of motivation.
- ☐ I tend to worry or feel anxious easily.
- ☐ I can get a little obsessive about things.
- ☐ Winter or long dark seasons lower my mood (seasonal affective disorder).
- ☐ I feel better after exercise—it lifts my mood noticeably.

Food & Cravings

- ☐ Chocolate gives me a mood boost.
- ☐ Cheese, wine, and chocolate are hard to resist—they make me feel better.
- ☐ Eating carbs temporarily improves my mood, but doesn't help my focus.

Focus & Behavior

- ☐ I've struggled with attention and focus since I was a kid.
- ☐ My motivation can feel low, even when I want to accomplish more.
- ☐ Addictive patterns (alcohol, smoking, or other habits) are easy for me to fall into.

Health History

- ☐ I live with chronic inflammation or an autoimmune condition (Graves', Hashimoto's, celiac, MS, etc.).
- ☐ I've experienced issues like fibromyalgia, constipation, or IBS.
- ☐ Inositol and 5-HTP help lift my mood.
- ☐ Lithium tends to make me feel worse, while SSRIs have actually helped.

GST / GPX "Detox & Defense" Self-Check

GST and GPX are part of your body's built-in detox and antioxidant defense system. Think of them as your internal clean-up crew, neutralizing toxins and keeping oxidative stress under control. When they're running sluggishly, your system can feel overloaded, like your "trash and recycling service" is always behind schedule.

Check off anything that resonates.

Environmental Sensitivity

- ☐ I'm sensitive to chemicals, fumes, or strong smells.
- ☐ I often feel better after sweating in a sauna or with a good workout.

☐ I have asthma, breathing difficulties, or often feel like I can't get enough air.
☐ I tend to feel tired, sluggish, or "toxic."

Health Patterns

☐ I developed gray or white hair earlier than most people my age.
☐ Stress brings on more gray hairs for me.
☐ I live with a chronic condition like asthma, eczema, psoriasis, autoimmune disease, diabetes, or inflammatory bowel disease.
☐ I experience chronic inflammation.
☐ I've fought off an infection recently, and it left me feeling drained.
☐ Neurological issues run in my personal or family history (tics, tremors, seizures, balance problems).

Weight & Metabolism

☐ I gain weight easily, even when I eat "the right foods."
☐ I have high blood pressure (or it runs in my family).
☐ Cancer is present in my family history.

NOS3 "Circulation & Resilience" Self-Check

NOS3 is a gene that helps your body make nitric oxide, the molecule that keeps your blood vessels flexible, your circulation strong, and your tissues well-nourished. When it's sluggish, blood flow and healing can take a hit.

Tick off the statements that sound like you.

Cardiovascular Signs

- ☐ My blood pressure tends to run higher than 120/80.
- ☐ I have a history of heart attack or atherosclerosis (plaque in the arteries).
- ☐ I had preeclampsia during pregnancy.
- ☐ I heal slowly after an injury or surgery.
- ☐ I notice swelling, sluggish circulation, or cold hands and feet.

Breathing & Energy

- ☐ I deal with asthma, chronic inflammation, or an autoimmune condition.
- ☐ I snore, breathe through my mouth, or have sleep apnea.
- ☐ I often feel low in energy or out of breath with minimal effort.

Hormones & Mood

- ☐ I am postmenopausal (or went through hormonal shifts that hit circulation hard).
- ☐ My moods swing up and down more than I'd like.
- ☐ I notice my memory isn't as sharp as it used to be.

Lifestyle Factors

- ☐ I don't move or exercise as much as I should.
- ☐ I live with chronic inflammation that affects my daily rhythm.
- ☐ I'm diabetic (type 1 or type 2).

PEMT "Liver & Cell Resilience" Self-Check

PEMT is a gene that helps your body make phosphatidylcholine, a critical building block for healthy cell membranes, fat metabolism, and liver detox. When it's under pressure, energy, mood, and digestion can all take a hit.

Mark the statements that sound familiar.

Body & Muscle Clues

- ☐ I deal with chronic, widespread muscle or body pain.
- ☐ I've been told I have fatty liver or trouble clearing fats.
- ☐ Fatty or greasy meals leave me feeling heavy or uncomfortable.

Nutrition & Lifestyle Patterns

- ☐ I'm vegetarian, vegan, or rarely eat foods rich in choline (like eggs, beef, organ meats, or caviar).
- ☐ I don't eat leafy greens very often.
- ☐ I've been diagnosed with small intestinal bacterial overgrowth (SIBO).

Hormones & Life Stages

- ☐ I am postmenopausal and know my estrogen is on the lower side.
- ☐ My symptoms began or worsened during/after pregnancy.
- ☐ Breastfeeding was physically or mentally depleting for me.

Medical & Family History

- ☐ I have gallstones or have had my gallbladder removed.
- ☐ My child was born with a congenital birth defect.

BHMT "Stress & Detox Pathway" Self-Check

BHMT is a key gene in your methylation cycle that helps recycle homocysteine, balance stress, and keep your liver and hormones working smoothly. When it's sluggish, energy, mood, and detox capacity often take a hit.

Check off what applies to you.

Mood & Mental Health

- ☐ I often feel anxious, irritable, or emotionally unstable.
- ☐ I have (or have had) depression.
- ☐ I experience mood swings or difficulty calming down after stress.
- ☐ I struggle with memory, focus, or brain fog.

Energy, Stress & Recovery

- ☐ I feel low in energy or "toxic" much of the time.
- ☐ I don't bounce back quickly after stress or illness.
- ☐ I get muscle aches or stiffness without a clear reason.
- ☐ I sweat very little, even with exercise or sauna use.

Digestion & Detox Clues

- ☐ I have difficulty digesting fats.
- ☐ I've had gallstones or had my gallbladder removed.
- ☐ I tend toward constipation, especially on high-fat or keto diets.
- ☐ I am sensitive to alcohol or don't tolerate it well.

- ☐ Choline-rich foods (like eggs, fish, or liver) don't always sit well with me.

Medical & Family History
- ☐ I have elevated homocysteine levels (if tested).
- ☐ I have elevated liver enzymes or fatty liver disease.
- ☐ I have a family history of heart disease or heart attack.

Hormones & Inflammation
- ☐ My estrogen levels are high, or I've experienced PMS/irregular cycles.
- ☐ I notice sluggish metabolism or stubborn weight gain.
- ☐ I have dry skin, eczema, or other skin irritations.
- ☐ I have a sulfur sensitivity (to foods like garlic, onions, crucifers).
- ☐ I feel worse when I take methylated B vitamins (methylfolate or methylcobalamin).

CBS "Sulfur Sensitivity & Detox Stress" Self-Check

CBS is a gene that helps break down sulfur-containing compounds. When it runs a little "fast" or is imbalanced, you can feel wired-but-tired, struggle with detox, and react to foods or supplements that others tolerate just fine.

Check what resonates with you.

Food & Supplement Sensitivities
- ☐ I react poorly to garlic, onions, eggs, broccoli, cabbage, or protein shakes.

- ☐ I feel worse after eating sulfur-rich veggies (like asparagus, kale, spinach, or cauliflower).
- ☐ I don't tolerate sulfur-based supplements (MSM, NAC, glutathione, alpha-lipoic acid).
- ☐ Methylated B vitamins make me feel worse instead of better.
- ☐ Alcohol doesn't sit well with me.

Energy & Body Clues

- ☐ I feel low in energy or fatigue that doesn't improve with rest.
- ☐ I feel sluggish or "toxic" after high-protein meals.
- ☐ My urine or sweat has a strong sulfur or ammonia-like odor.
- ☐ I often feel wired but tired, especially in the evening.
- ☐ I notice headaches, migraines, or body aches without a clear cause.

Mood & Brain

- ☐ I experience brain fog or mental fatigue.
- ☐ I have a hard time focusing and concentrating.
- ☐ I feel anxious, irritable, or overstimulated.
- ☐ I experience ADD/ADHD-like symptoms.
- ☐ Sleep can be a struggle—either falling asleep or staying asleep.

Detox & Environmental Reactions

- ☐ I feel worse after detox practices (sauna, Epsom salt bath, heavy sweating).

- ☐ I've had histamine or mast cell-type reactions (rashes, flushing, congestion).
- ☐ I am sensitive to chemicals, fragrances, or strong odors.
- ☐ Bright light or screen glare makes my eyes feel strained.
- ☐ I get random heart palpitations or a racing heartbeat without explanation.

MTR "B12, Folate & Energy Metabolism" Self-Check

The MTR gene helps recycle folate and vitamin B12, two nutrients that keep your brain sharp, your energy steady, and your detox pathways humming. When it's sluggish, you might feel drained, foggy, or stressed out more easily.

Check what feels true for you.

Energy & Motivation

- ☐ I feel tired, sluggish, or "drained" most days.
- ☐ I crave sugar or carbs to get through the day.
- ☐ I have low motivation or feel apathetic.
- ☐ I wake up feeling unrested, or I struggle to get good sleep.
- ☐ I often feel wired but exhausted, especially in the afternoons.

Mood & Brain Function

- ☐ I have a history of depression, mood swings, or anxiety.
- ☐ I experience nervousness or panic attacks.
- ☐ I struggle with brain fog or slow processing.
- ☐ My memory and concentration aren't as sharp as I'd like.
- ☐ I feel easily overwhelmed or unable to handle stress well.

Nerves & Circulation

- ☐ I experience numbness, tingling, or "pins and needles."
- ☐ I get lightheaded or dizzy when standing up quickly.
- ☐ I have a family history of stroke, heart disease, or neurological disorders.
- ☐ I've been told my homocysteine levels are high (if tested).
- ☐ I notice headaches or migraines are a regular issue.

Nutrient Clues

- ☐ I've had low B12 levels, even when supplementing.
- ☐ I don't tolerate folic acid well.
- ☐ I feel worse on methylated B vitamins (methylcobalamin, methylfolate).
- ☐ I do better with hydroxy- or adenosyl-B12.
- ☐ I have a history of being vegan or vegetarian without consistent B12 support.

Body Signals

- ☐ I get frequent mouth sores or ulcers.
- ☐ I have skin issues like eczema or dermatitis.
- ☐ My digestion feels "off"—bloating, IBS, or poor nutrient absorption.
- ☐ I've noticed I recover poorly from stress, illness, or overexertion.
- ☐ I feel sensitive to perfumes, smoke, or environmental chemicals.

SHMT "Folate, Gut, and Repair" Self-Check

The SHMT gene plays a central role in folate metabolism, DNA repair, and gut balance. When it's sluggish, you may notice fertility challenges, low energy, gut issues, and poor recovery.

Check what resonates with you.

Energy & Brain Function

- ☐ I have low energy or fatigue that doesn't improve with rest.
- ☐ I have poor memory, brain fog, or mental sluggishness.
- ☐ I find it hard to focus or concentrate.
- ☐ I feel nutrient-depleted even when eating well.
- ☐ I feel overwhelmed or worse when taking folate or methylated B vitamins.

Fertility & Reproduction

- ☐ I have a history of miscarriages.
- ☐ I've given birth to a baby with low birth weight.
- ☐ My child has a congenital birth defect.
- ☐ I have fertility struggles or trouble conceiving.
- ☐ I've had anemia or borderline low hemoglobin despite iron supplementation.
- ☐ There's a family history of miscarriage or neural tube defects.

Gut & Digestion

- ☐ I've been diagnosed with SIBO (small intestinal bacterial overgrowth).
- ☐ I experience frequent bloating, gas, or food sensitivities.

- ☐ I feel worse on high-protein diets.
- ☐ I don't respond well to synthetic folic acid.
- ☐ My digestion and nutrient absorption feel compromised.

Immunity & Recovery

- ☐ I get sick easily and take a long time to recover.
- ☐ My wounds heal slowly or poorly.
- ☐ I notice poor recovery after illness, injury, or physical stress.
- ☐ I have a family history of autoimmune conditions.

Hormones & Skin

- ☐ I have hormonal imbalances (PMS, irregular cycles, or low progesterone).
- ☐ I have skin issues like rashes, acne, or a dull complexion.
- ☐ I experience irritability or mood swings related to digestion or diet.
- ☐ I've struggled with insomnia or disrupted sleep.
- ☐ I have or have had depression.

My score:

MTHFR ___	NOS3 ___
DAO ___	PEMT ___
COMT (slow) ___	BHMT ___
COMT (fast) ___	CBS ___
MAOA (slow) ___	MTR ___
MAOA (fast) ___	SHMT ___
GST/GPX ___	

Scoring:

0 points: Excellent! This gene looks strong, balanced, and functioning smoothly.

1–4 points: Great work—this gene may need a little fine-tuning, but most of the challenges likely come from other genes.

5–7 points: This gene could use some extra care. Follow the daily prompts to help restore balance.

8+ points: This gene is struggling and needs focused attention to clean up.

Follow the prompts in this book, then reassess yourself using the other assessment and notice how many of your symptoms have eased or even disappeared.

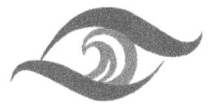

Inflamed, Exhausted, or Anxious? Let's Talk Stress

Before you proceed with the next two assessments, I want to talk a little more about stress, mindset, and spirituality. As we have already discussed in the Blue Zones section, stress, mindset, and connection to family and community are very important for longevity and health.

Stress . . . let's face it, we cannot escape it, but we also know that not all stress is bad. Some stress is actually good for us. Good stress (eustress) vs. bad stress (distress) helps you recognize which pressure is helping you grow and which is silently burning you out, accelerating your aging process, and literally killing you. Are you getting the point?!

Good Stress (Eustress)

This is the motivating, short-term kind of stress that pushes you to rise to a challenge, grow, and build resilience.

Examples of good stress:
- Starting a new job or project you're excited about
- Giving a speech or performance
- Physical exercise (when balanced)

- Studying for an exam that leads to a goal
- Moving to a new city for a fresh opportunity
- Healthy deadlines that keep you focused

Think of good stress as a stretch that feels so good, not a painful strain. It may be uncomfortable, but it energizes and motivates you.

Bad Stress (Distress)

This is the overwhelming, chronic, or unresolved stress that drains your energy, disrupts health, and can trigger anxiety, burnout, disease, or even death—YEP!

Examples of bad stress:
- Staying in a toxic relationship or environment
- Financial instability with no support
- Chronic sleep deprivation
- Long-term caregiving without respite
- Being overworked and undervalued
- Constant worry or rumination
- Trauma (unresolved emotional pain)
- Physical illness with no treatment plan
- Daily overwhelm from decision fatigue or multitasking

Bad stress feels like you are stuck between a rock and a hard place. It's often prolonged, heavy pressure without a purpose and without a clear end in sight.

KEY DIFFERENCE:

	Good Stress	Bad Stress
Duration	Short-term	Long-term or chronic
Effect	Motivating, energizing	Draining, anxiety-producing
Outcome	Personal growth, achievement	Burnout, health problems
Perception	"I can handle this"	"I'm drowning in this"

Now that we know that there is good and bad stress, let's take a look at the stress we create ourselves compared to the stress that is out of our control.

1. Self-created (or perceived) stress—also known as the worst kind of stress, the do-it-to-yourself kind of stress

This is the stress we generate internally and often unintentionally. It's rooted in our thoughts, beliefs, habits, perfectionism, fears, or the stories we tell ourselves. I really want you to take note of the word PERCEIVED, as this is the key word in the stress we create ourselves. I will give you tools to help you check in with yourself and see if your stress is "real" or *perceived*.

Examples:
- Overthinking worst-case scenarios
- Trying to please everyone

- Obsessing over the future
- Judging yourself harshly
- Holding yourself to impossible standards
- Comparing yourself to others on social media
- Creating urgency where none truly exists

Your body reacts to imagined danger the same way it does to real danger. So, even if there's no physical threat, your nervous system stays in fight-or-flight mode with elevated cortisol, shallow breathing, tension, poor digestion, and poor sleep. Most chronic anxiety, burnout, and inflammation are tied to this self-created stress loop. *Remember this paragraph because this is also how you will change your life!*

2. Uncontrollable (external) stress—also known as bad stress

This includes situations outside of your immediate influence; real challenges that life throws your way.

Examples:
- A family member's illness
- A sudden job loss
- Global events, economic uncertainty
- Natural disasters
- Past trauma resurfacing
- Health diagnoses

Even though you can't control these situations, you can control your response to them, and that determines how deeply they impact your long-term health. This is the life-changing stuff that I am talking about.

Are you ready to go really deep, like mind-blowing, life-changing deep? Let's do a deeper dive by answering a few more assessments to see how much stress you have or still carry from your past and how strong your mindset is!

Mental Health: Adverse Childhood Experiences (ACEs) Assessment

This questionnaire is intended for adults (18 years or older). Please check all that apply to you, then add up the number of checked boxes to determine your ACE score. Allocate one point to each answer.

Due to the personal nature of these questions, you may choose not to share your responses with your healthcare provider. Instead, you may choose to share only your final ACE score.

Psychological Abuse

- ☐ Did a parent or other adult often swear at you, insult you, put you down, or humiliate you?
- ☐ Did a parent or other adult often act in a way that made you afraid that you might be physically hurt?

Physical Abuse

- ☐ Did a parent or other adult often push, grab, slap, or throw something at you?
- ☐ Did a parent or other adult often hit you so hard that you had marks or were injured?

Sexual Abuse

- ☐ Did an adult or person at least five years older than you ever touch you inappropriately or fondle you?

- ☐ Did an adult or a person at least five years older than you ask you to touch their body in an inappropriate way?

- ☐ Did an adult or a person at least five years older than you attempt to have or actually have oral, anal, or vaginal sex with you?

Substance Abuse

- ☐ Did you live with or spend a lot of time with anyone who was a problem drinker or alcoholic?

- ☐ Did you live with or spend a lot of time with anyone who used illicit drugs recreationally or habitually?

Neglect

- ☐ Did you regularly experience a lack of access to food, clothing, shelter, or medical care when it was needed?

- ☐ Did you regularly experience a lack of affection, companionship, or support from your parents, household members, or primary caregivers?

- ☐ Were you regularly left unsupervised or minimally supervised for long periods of time?

- ☐ Did your parents or primary caregivers regularly express a lack of interest or concern about your whereabouts or friendships?

- ☐ Did you regularly experience a lack of interaction (e.g., play, bedtime reading, help with homework, etc.) with your parents or primary caregivers?

Mental Illness in the Household

- ☐ Did a parent, household member, or primary caregiver have depression or another mood disorder, or any type of mental illness?
- ☐ Did a parent, household member, close family member, or primary caregiver attempt suicide?

Parental Relationships

- ☐ Did your parents or other family members often shout, fight, or exchange physical blows with one another?
- ☐ Were your parents ever separated or divorced?
- ☐ Was your mother or stepmother sometimes or often pushed, grabbed, or slapped? Did she sometimes or often have objects thrown at her?
- ☐ Was your mother or stepmother sometimes or often kicked, bitten, hit with a fist, or hit with something hard?
- ☐ Was your mother or stepmother ever hit repeatedly for several minutes?
- ☐ Was your mother or stepmother ever threatened with or hurt by a knife or gun?

Criminal Behavior in the Household

- ☐ Did a parent or household member regularly engage in illegal activities or behaviors?
- ☐ Did a parent or household member ever go to prison?

Total:_____

Interpreting Your ACE Score

Your ACE score is an indicator of exposure to significant stressors and trauma during childhood. ACEs are relatively common. In fact, most people report an ACE score of at least 1. In general, higher ACE scores are associated with an increased risk for diabetes, cancer, depression, anxiety, and alcohol or drug abuse as an adult.

Research indicates that individuals who are more resilient are less likely to experience the long-term effects of ACEs. Your functional medicine provider can offer you many tools, such as cognitive behavioral therapy, meditation, and other mindfulness-based practices, that can help to increase your resilience and reduce the impact of ACEs on your health and well-being.

Perceived Stress Assessment

For each question, choose from the following alternatives:

0 = never

1 = almost never

2 = sometimes

3 = fairly often

4 = very often

1. In the last month, how often have you been upset because of something that happened unexpectedly?
2. In the last month, how often have you felt that you were unable to control the important things in your life?
3. In the past month, how often have you felt nervous and stressed?

4. In the past month, how often have you felt confident about your ability to handle your personal problems?
5. In the past month, how often have you felt that things were going your way?
6. In the past month, how often have you found that you could not cope with all the things that you had to do?
7. In the past month, how often have you been able to control irritations in your life?
8. In the past month, how often have you felt that you were on top of things?
9. In the past month, how often have you been angered because of things that happened that were outside of your control?
10. In the past month, how often have you felt that difficulties were piling up so high that you could not overcome them?

Figuring out your PSA Score

First, you need to reverse your score on questions 4, 5, 7, and 8. For these four questions, 0 = 4, 1 = 3, 2 = 2, and 4 = 0. Then add up your score from each question to get the total.

Total _____

Scores can range from 0 to 40, with higher scores indicating higher perceived stress.

Scores ranging from 0 to 13 would be considered low stress.

Scores ranging from 14 to 26 would be considered moderate stress.

Scores ranging from 27 to 40 would be considered high perceived stress.

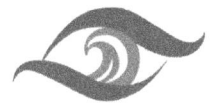

Eat Like You Love Yourself; Move Like You Mean It

Nourishing your body with the proper food and adding lots of movement to each day will enhance circulation, support lymphatic drainage and detoxification, and boost collagen and elastin, giving your skin that firm, glowing resilience we all want. You'll also strengthen muscle, tone your body, fuel your mind, improve digestion, and support hormone balance, as well as reduce inflammation, smooth fine lines, reverse signs of aging, and promote healthy weight management.

What Your Plate Should Look Like:

- Whole, unprocessed, nutrient-dense foods
- Lean proteins (plant or animal)
- Healthy fats (avocado, olive oil, nuts, seeds)
- Slow-digesting, fiber-rich carbohydrates (like sweet potatoes, quinoa, or legumes)
- A colorful variety of vegetables
- Herbs and spices that promote healing (like turmeric, ginger, cinnamon)

Choose wild-caught seafood when possible because it's higher in omega-3s and free of toxins. For meats and poultry, prioritize pasture-raised, grass-fed, grass-finished, and organic. These options are richer in nutrients and free from synthetic hormones and antibiotics that can disrupt your hormonal balance and inflammation pathways.

80/20 Lifestyle Rule: Just like we aim to eat until 80% full, think of your lifestyle as 80% intentional, and 20% flexible fun. This isn't about being perfect; it's about being consistent and kind to yourself. Really, really enjoy that 20%, guilt-free.

Protein First

Protein is essential; it's the building block of your body. It fuels muscle growth, supports energy, and plays a key role in cellular regeneration and fat metabolism.

Goals:

- Minimum: 30g of protein per meal
- Ideal: Your target body weight in grams of protein per day (for example, if your ideal weight is 135 lbs, aim for 135g/day)

Animal protein sources are more bioavailable, meaning your body absorbs more of them. If you're plant-based, you'll need slightly more to get the same effect. For example, if you eat 30g of animal protein, you'll need 33–37g of plant protein to match the absorption. Also, remember that not all plant proteins are complete. Pair them wisely (e.g., rice + beans, hummus + pita, lentils + quinoa) to ensure you're getting all the essential amino acids.

Macronutrient Strategy

- Prioritize protein first.
- Adjust carbs and fats based on your personal energy demands and lifestyle.
- Stay flexible, not rigid.

Please avoid fake meats. If you can't pronounce even one of the ingredients on the label, your body can't process them either.

If you need help crafting meals that will nourish your body and movement specifically designed to support youthful vitality, radiant energy, and deep cellular repair, I offer a membership program (more info is available at the end of the book). The nutrient-dense meals are crafted to enhance circulation, support lymphatic drainage and detoxification, and boost collagen and elastin, giving your skin that firm, glowing resilience we all want. You'll also strengthen muscle, tone your body, and fuel your mind. In short, you're about to glow from the inside out.

Each meal is an opportunity to nourish your body on a cellular level. The foods you'll eat will be anti-inflammatory, rich in essential nutrients, healthy fats, lean protein, and fiber.

The Migrating Motor Complex (MMC)

Now let's talk digestion. Your body has a natural cleaning system between meals called the Migrating Motor Complex (MMC). Think of it like a little train that clears out the digestive tract.

Imagine you have a little train that lives inside your stomach, and when you eat in the morning, the train gets filled up with all the food you just ate, and then it gets on its way. It needs time to go through a lot of intestines to process everything and to allow your body to absorb the nutrients it needs before it heads back to the stomach to pick up the next meal.

But if you eat before the train has dropped everything off, the body signals for the train to come back up to the stomach ASAP to catch the food you are currently eating. What do you think happens to all the previous food that was still on the train and is now covered by the new food? It rots and ferments, so even if you choose healthy, nutrient-dense foods, it doesn't matter because your body cannot process them.

It kicks in every three to four hours after you eat, but it only works if you're not snacking. If you eat again before the train finishes its route, the body hits the panic button, calls the train back, and now food piles on top of food...fermentation, bloating, poor absorption—you get the picture.

Key MMC Guidelines:
- Leave three to four hours between meals.
- Avoid snacking and eat meals that keep you satiated.
- If you're hungry, drink water first, as thirst often disguises itself as hunger.
- Stop eating at least three hours before bed.
- Ideal eating window: 8 a.m.–5 p.m.

Let's Talk Fasting

Fasting isn't just a trend; it's a biologically programmed repair mechanism. Benefits include:

- Improved blood sugar regulation

- Increased fat-burning and metabolic flexibility
- Cellular repair via autophagy
- Hormonal balance
- Reduced inflammation
- Enhanced brain clarity and focus

But here's the thing . . . fasting affects men and women differently. While men often thrive with extended fasts, women (especially those cycling) need a gentler approach to avoid hormone disruption. I am not saying that a woman should never do a longer type of fast; there are definitely benefits to it, but we need to fast wisely and according to our cycle.

Ideal Practice for Women:
- Eat between 8 a.m. and 5 p.m.
- Fast between 5 p.m. and 8 a.m. (15 hours)
- Your body starts "fasting" three hours after your last meal, so stopping earlier really matters!
- Sync deeper fasts with the right time of your cycle for maximum benefit (we'll talk more about this soon).

You're not just starting a "diet," you're starting a vitality transformation. You're going to feel clearer, more energized, and more aligned mentally, emotionally, physically, and spiritually.

Ready?

Let's go!

Here are the benefits of the different lengths of fasts[6]:

Intermittent Fasting: 12-16 hours:
- Helps you lose weight
- Improves focus & concentration
- Boosts energy levels

Autophagy Fasting: 17-72 hours:
- Detoxes the body
- Improves brain function & cognition
- Prevents colds
- Balances sex hormones

Gut Rest Fast: 24+ hours:
- Counteracts antibiotic use
- Offsets birth control use
- Helps with SIBO

Fat Burn Fast: 36+ hours:
- Minimizes weight loss resistance
- Releases stored sugar
- Reduces cholesterol

Dopamine Reset Fast: 48+ hours:
- Reboots dopamine levels
- Lowers anxiety levels

---

[6] Dr. Mindy Pelz, *Fast like a Girl* (US: Hay House, 2023) pgs. 29-39.

Immune Reset Fast: 72+ hours:

- Eases chronic conditions
- Prevents chronic diseases
- Alleviates pain & stiffness from musculoskeletal injuries that won't go away
- Slows down the effects of aging

Here is the important thing: once you've broken your fast, the order in which you eat your food matters more than you think. Why? Because it dramatically affects your blood sugar response, and keeping glucose stable is everything when it comes to energy, mood, weight, inflammation, and long-term health.

Here's Your Ideal Eating Order:

1. Fiber first (a handful of greens, cucumbers, carrots, flax, chia)
2. Proteins and fats next (chicken, salmon, eggs, avocado, olive oil)
3. Then starches and carbs (sweet potatoes, rice, quinoa, bread)
4. Sugars last (dessert, fruit, wine)

I'm not saying you need to completely finish eating each group before moving to the next. You don't have to finish your broccoli before you're "allowed" to eat your salmon. But start with a few bites of fiber, layer in some protein and fat, and save the carbs and sugars for later in the meal.

Let me paint you a picture. If you eat in the order I just shared, fiber → protein/fat → carbs → sugar, your blood sugar will rise gently, let's say, only to the height of a school bus. Manageable, steady, and easy for your body to handle. Then, over the next two hours, it will slowly come back down. Controlled, stable, calm.

But if you eat sugar first or even wait an hour after dinner for dessert, your glucose will go from a flat line straight to the top of the Burj Khalifa (you know, the tallest building in the world) and then crash hard over the following two hours. And then you wonder why you feel fatigue, irritability, brain fog, cravings, and have long-term health damage.

Consistently allowing your glucose to spike and crash like that increases the risk of:

- Insulin resistance
- Type 2 diabetes
- Heart disease
- Kidney damage
- Nerve damage
- Eye disease

I don't want to scare you, but this is serious. If eating a few carrots before your pizza helps avoid all that, isn't it worth it?

Just to prove to you how much sugar affects you and just how addictive it is, I want to share one more powerful (and horrifying) study with you. Harvard researchers took mice and got them addicted to cocaine. Then, they placed two water bottles in their cage: One was laced with cocaine and the other was laced with sugar.

Guess what happened? The *already* cocaine-addicted mice chose sugar over and over again. Sugar was found to be up to eight times more addictive than cocaine.[7] Let that sink in. And yet sugar is on every shelf, at a child's eye level, in colorful packaging, completely legal and totally normalized.

I know it's hard to quit. Knowing what to eat is one thing, but actually doing it, especially when your brain is chemically hooked on sugar, is another story.

A Few Tips to Help You Break Free from Sugar

Here are some small shifts that make a huge difference:

- Drink water when you're craving sugar; it's often dehydration in disguise.
- Never shop hungry. Just don't do it.
- Avoid the aisles. The real food lives around the perimeter of the store—produce, meat, seafood, and eggs. The aisles are filled with processed stuff designed to hook you.

SWAP OUT	FOR[8]
Coffee or black tea	Green or oolong tea
Bananas	Berries
Potatoes	Beets, kohlrabi, carrots, or sweet potatoes

---

[7] Rachel Dvoskin, "Sweeter than Cocaine," Scientific American, February 20, 2024, https://www.scientificamerican.com/article/sweeter-than-cocaine/?utm_source=chatgpt.com.

[8] Kara N. Fitzgerald, *Younger You: Reduce Your Bio Age and Live Longer* (Solon, OH: Findaway World, LLC, 2022).

Typical Hamburgers	Grass-fed burgers, wild-caught salmon burgers
Vegetable oil, soybean oil, cottonseed oil, canola oil, grapeseed oil, safflower oil (for cooking)	Avocado oil, coconut oil, MCT oil
Regular olive oil	Organic, extra virgin olive oil, bonus points for rosemary-infused (only for drizzling on salads and cooked foods. Don't cook with it).
Potato chips and other bagged snacks	Roasted beet chips, roasted chick peas, seaweed snacks, kale chips, plantain chips, sunflower seeds, pumpkin seeds
Hot chocolate	Turmeric-rich golden milk
Pasta	Quinoa, legumes, pasta
Sausage	Sauteed shiitake mushrooms, or if you want a real sausage, get a clean-sourced product, fresh organic chicken, grass-fed, and grass-finished
Iceberg or regular lettuce	Spinach, arugula, kale, chard, and collard greens as a base for the salad
White or brown sugar	Stevia, monk fruit, inulin, erythritol, honey, maple syrup
Peanut butter	Almond butter, sunflower butter, pumpkin seed butter, baruka butter
Cereal	Grain-free, nut and seed-heavy granola, porridge made from quinoa, eggs

Conventional produce and meat	Organic produce, meat that is pasture-raised or grass-fed whenever possible, fish that is wild caught or third-party verified, clean farm-raised
White bread	Sprouted grain bread, Himalayan tartary buckwheat flour
Candy	Dark chocolate (70%+), dates with nut butter
Regular milk	Unsweetened almond, cashew, or coconut milk
Flavored yogurts	Plain Greek yogurt or coconut yogurt with fresh fruit
Factory-farmed eggs	Pasture-raised, organic eggs
Ketchup & BBQ sauce	Homemade salsa, mustard, tahini, avocado mash
Store-bought salad dressings	Olive oil + lemon or balsamic + herbs or any other homemade dressing with healthy oils
Store-bought muffins & pastries	Homemade almond flour muffins or protein bites
Ice cream	Blended frozen banana "nice cream" with nut butter or cacao
Pudding	Chia seed pudding with coconut milk and berries
Cookies	Himalayan tartary buckwheat flour, homemade oat or coconut flour cookies with natural sweeteners like honey or monk fruit

Eat the Rainbow, Literally! (Skittles NOT Included)

Fruits and vegetables get their colors from phytonutrients, powerful plant compounds that protect and nourish your cells. Each color signals a different group of nutrients and healing benefits, which is why you want at least one from each color group daily.

RED

Nutrients: Lycopene, anthocyanins, vitamin C

Benefits:
- Reduces heart disease risk
- Supports prostate & breast health
- Potent antioxidants (free radical defense)

ORANGE

Nutrients: Beta-carotene, vitamin C, flavonoids

Benefits:
- Boosts immunity
- Supports skin & eye health
- Lowers inflammation

YELLOW

Nutrients: Lutein, zeaxanthin, vitamin C

Benefits:
- Supports vision
- Enhances skin glow
- Aids digestion and immune strength

GREEN

Nutrients: Chlorophyll, folate, vitamin K, sulforaphane

Benefits:

- Detoxifies the liver
- Supports bones, brain, and hormones
- Promotes healthy aging

PURPLE / BLUE

Nutrients: Anthocyanins, resveratrol, flavonoids

Benefits:

- Protects memory and cognition
- Cardiovascular support
- Anti-aging and anti-inflammatory

WHITE / BROWN

Nutrients: Allicin, quercetin, potassium, fiber

Benefits:

- Boosts immune function
- Lowers blood pressure
- Supports heart health and inflammation

Daily Rainbow Cheat Sheet

To make this simple: Aim for nine servings of fruits and veggies per day, including at least one from each color. Below this section, you'll find a color-coded checklist, a simple daily tracker to help you hit your phytonutrient goals and truly eat the rainbow. Use it, enjoy it, and watch what happens to your energy, skin, mood, and clarity over time.

Phytonutrient Spectrum Checklist

RED		
Foods	**Weekly Servings**	**Benefits**
Apples, Beans (adzuki, kidney, red), Beets, Bell peppers, Blood oranges, Cranberries, Cherries, Grapefruit (pink), Goji berries, Grapes, Guava, Onions, Plums, Pomegranate, Potatoes, Prickly pear, Radicchio, Radishes, Raspberries, Strawberries, Sweet red peppers, Rhubarb, Rooibos tea, Tomato, Watermelon	☐ SUN ☐ MON ☐ TUES ☐ WED ☐ THURS ☐ FRI ☐ SAT	Anti-bacterial, Anti-cancer, Anti-inflammatory, Blood vessel health, Brain health, Cell protection, Heart health, Prostate health
ORANGE		
Foods	**Weekly Servings**	**Benefits**
Apricots, Bell peppers, Cantaloupe, Carrots, Mango, Nectarine, Orange, Papaya, Persimmons, Pumpkin, Squash (acorn, buttercup, butternut, winter), Sweet potato, Tangerines, Turmeric root, Yams	☐ SUN ☐ MON ☐ TUES ☐ WED ☐ THURS ☐ FRI ☐ SAT	Anti-inflammatory, Blood vessel health, Brain health, Cell protection, Heart health, Reproductive health

YELLOW

Foods	Weekly Servings	Benefits
Apple, Asian pears, Banana, Bell peppers, Ginger root, Jackfruit, Lemon, Millet, Passionfruit, Pineapple, Plantains, Starfruit, Summer squash	☐ SUN ☐ MON ☐ TUES ☐ WED ☐ THURS ☐ FRI ☐ SAT	Anti-inflammatory, Cell protection, Digestive health, Eye health, Heart health, Immune health

GREEN

Foods	Weekly Servings	Benefits
Apples, Artichoke, Asparagus, Avocado, Bamboo sprouts, Bean sprouts, Bitter melon, Bok choy, Broccoli, Broccolini, Brussels sprouts, Cabbage, Celery, Chayote, Cucumbers, Feijoa, Green beans, Green peas, decaf Green tea, Greens (arugula, chard, collard, kale, mustard, spinach, turnip), Kiwi, Limes, Nopales, Okra, Olives, Pears, Snow peas, Tomatillos, Watercress, Zucchini	☐ SUN ☐ MON ☐ TUES ☐ WED ☐ THURS ☐ FRI ☐ SAT	Anti-cancer, Anti-inflammatory, Blood vessel health, Bone health, Brain health, Cell protection, Heart health, Hormone balance, Metabolic health

BLUE/PURPLE/BLACK

Foods	Weekly Servings	Benefits
Bell peppers, Berries (blue, black, boysenberries, huckleberries, marionberries), Cabbage, Carrots, Cauliflower, Eggplant, Figs, Grapes, Kale, Olives, Plums, Potatoes, Prunes, Raisins, Rice (black or purple)	☐ SUN ☐ MON ☐ TUES ☐ WED ☐ THURS ☐ FRI ☐ SAT	Anti-inflammatory, Blood vessel health, Bone health, Brain health, Cell protection, Digestive health, Heart health, Liver health

WHITE/TAN/BROWN

Foods	Weekly Servings	Benefits
Apples, Applesauce, Bean dips, Cassava (yuca root), Cauliflower, Cherimoya, Coconut, Dates, Garlic, Ginger, Jicama, Legumes (chickpeas, dried beans or peas, hummus, lentils, peanuts, refried beans/low-fat), Lychee, Mushrooms, Nuts (almonds, cashews, pecans, walnuts), Onions, Pears, Pitaya (dragon fruit), Sauerkraut, Seeds (flax, hemp, pumpkin, sesame, sunflower), Shallots, Tahini, Taro root, Turnips, Naturally caffeine free tea (black, white), Gluten-free whole grains (amaranth, brown rice, quinoa, teff)	☐ SUN ☐ MON ☐ TUES ☐ WED ☐ THURS ☐ FRI ☐ SAT	Anti-cancer, Anti-inflammatory, Blood vessel health, Bone health, Brain health, Cell protection, Digestive health, Heart health, Immune health, Metabolic health

1. We want at least nine servings of whole plant food per day to prevent chronic disease (and remember prevention is better than cure!) A serving is
   - ½ cup of cooked veggies
   - 1 cup of raw leafy veggies
   - Medium-sized piece of fruit
   - Do your best to have three servings at each meal.

2. Instead of eating your standard American breakfast, which tends to be white and brown (seriously, think about it—pancakes, waffles, toast, bagels, cereals that are colored with all kinds of dyes), I dare you to try something different tomorrow morning.

   One option might be a rainbow smoothie—add blueberries, peaches, raspberries, and a handful of dark leafy greens, and you already have four of the nine colors you are meant to eat in a day. Add a little bit of protein powder (my favorite is Be Well By Kelly grass-fed beef protein powder, or she also has a plant-based one), a scoop of creatine, and Bob's your uncle!

3. There are thousands of phytonutrients in nature, so make sure you are not stuck eating the same 10 foods, even if you are getting all the colors in. I once heard one of my professors say that we are meant to eat 50 different fruits and veggies in one week and 200 different plants in one month. That is a lot of variety!

   While variety is extremely important, for now, introduce one new plant food per week. Go on, give it a go! You just might find your new favorite food!

4. Food synergy refers to the powerful interactions between nutrients in different foods that enhance their absorption, effectiveness, or health benefits. Here are some delicious examples:

- Turmeric + black pepper + healthy fat (e.g., olive oil)

    Why it works: Curcumin (the active compound in turmeric) has low bioavailability on its own. Piperine in black pepper enhances absorption by up to 2,000%, and fat (such as olive oil or avocado) helps dissolve and transport curcumin.

- Spinach (iron) + lemon (vitamin C)

    Why it works: Non-heme iron in plants like spinach is poorly absorbed, but vitamin C converts it into a more absorbable form. A squeeze of lemon or pairing with bell peppers dramatically boosts iron bioavailability.

- Tomatoes + avocado or olive oil

    Why it works: Lycopene (a potent antioxidant in tomatoes) is fat-soluble. Pairing with healthy fats enhances absorption; think: caprese salad with olive oil or guacamole with salsa.

- Carrots + olive oil or nut butters

    Why it works: Beta-carotene (a precursor to vitamin A) is also fat-soluble. Adding a fat source such as olive oil, tahini, or almond butter helps your body absorb it more efficiently.

- Oats (beta-glucan) + berries (polyphenols)

    Why it works: The soluble fiber in oats slows glucose absorption, and polyphenols in berries support gut health and reduce oxidative stress. Together, they enhance metabolic and cardiovascular benefits.

- Eggs + salad greens

    Why it works: The fat and protein in eggs significantly increase absorption of carotenoids like lutein and zeaxanthin from leafy greens, a key ingredient for eye and skin health.

- Garlic + fish (omega-3s)

    Why it works: Garlic may enhance the anti-inflammatory and cardiovascular effects of omega-3 fatty acids, and together they support healthy lipid profiles and reduce blood pressure.

- Beans (zinc/iron) + onions/garlic (sulfur compounds)

    Why it works: Allium compounds in garlic and onions improve mineral absorption from plant foods, particularly zinc and iron, making vegan meals more nutrient-rich.

Lastly, I wanted to add that no matter how good you are with your diet, if you are still not losing weight or if your symptoms are not reducing, you should also consider food intolerances and food allergies.

You can do a blood test, and I have a favorite lab that does it, Cyrex Labs. You can also do a 10- to 14-day diet diary. In one column, write what time you are eating, in the next column write what you are eating (don't be perfect all of a sudden, this isn't a judgment, this is to try and connect the dots), and in the third column, write how you are feeling and at what time you started feeling it.

The reason you want to know this is that there are a few types of food reactions. IgE is when you have a reaction to a food within minutes to hours. This includes anaphylaxis, but it doesn't have to be that severe. With this type of reaction, you should stop eating this food, period.

There is such a thing as microdosing, but for the sake of this book, I suggest you stop eating the food that gives you a reaction within minutes of eating it.

Next is the IgG reaction, which is a food intolerance, and this reaction can occur within hours to days, typically four hours to 72 days. So if you eat a tomato on Monday and on Wednesday you get a headache, you might not see the clear line, but if you are getting headaches within hours to days of eating tomatoes, another one after you ate an eggplant, another one after you had some peppers, you might be able to see that you have an intolerance to foods in the nightshade family.

For this type of reaction, I would take out the food you are reacting to for four weeks and then slowly start introducing it again, every four days, and wait to see if there is still a reaction.

If you have skin issues, eliminate allergens for six weeks, as that's how long it takes for the skin to fully heal. Then you can start testing one food at a time every four days.

If you'd like to go deeper into this topic and get help with the elimination diet, feel free to contact my office or set up an appointment with a Functional Medicine doctor near you!

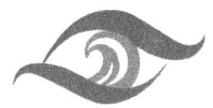

The Monthly Map: Eat, Move, and Thrive With Your Hormones

For the Ladies (and Actually Men too, You All Have at Least One Female in Your Life—Pay Attention!)

Let's talk cycle syncing, and if you're a man reading this, don't scroll past. Understanding the rhythm of the female body can transform your relationships, deepen empathy, and maybe even prevent a few unnecessary arguments.

Cycle syncing is a method of aligning your diet, exercise, and lifestyle with the natural hormonal shifts that occur during a woman's menstrual cycle. When you tune into these phases rather than push against them, you unlock:

- Better energy
- Improved hormone balance
- Enhanced fitness results
- Reduced stress and fatigue
- Elevated mood and mental clarity

It's about working with your body, not against it.

Why Cycle Syncing Matters After 40

As we age, hormone levels shift, and so does the body's ability to maintain lean muscle mass, especially post-40. Muscle isn't just about tone or aesthetics; it's a longevity organ. It supports everything from metabolism and joint health to immune function and mental well-being.

That's why this plan focuses less on weight loss and more on muscle growth, hormone harmony, and sustainable health.

- On strength training days: Do not fast. You need fuel to build muscle and support recovery. Prioritize protein and nutrient-dense meals around workouts to feed your muscles.
- Strength + stretch = longevity: Building muscle is only half the equation. Flexibility, mobility, and fascia support are equally important, especially as we age. Balance your strength work with stretching, pilates, yoga, and fascia release throughout the month.
- Each phase of your cycle calls for different movement and food; we'll guide you through how to eat, train, and recover in a way that respects your body's unique rhythm.

This isn't just about looking fit. It's about feeling strong, vibrant, and balanced in your skin all month long and all life long. The more you understand your body's fluctuations and work with them, the more energy, resilience, and power you'll unlock.

So yes, ladies, your body has seasons every single month. And fellas, if you're still reading, knowing this? Game changer.

Four Phases

Menstrual Phase: The start of the cycle, where the uterine lining sheds (period).

Follicular Phase: Hormones rise as the body prepares for ovulation; energy and mood improve.

Ovulation Phase: The release of an egg, when fertility peaks and energy is highest.

Luteal Phase: Hormones shift as the body prepares for menstruation again, and cravings or mood changes may occur.

PHASE 1—Menstruation: Days 1-7

Top Tips:

- Focus inward & release what is not serving you.
- Reconnect with your inner self.
- Breathwork and restorative yoga to downshift your nervous system.
- Earlier bedtimes to allow deep tissue repair.

Diet:

- Follow a dairy-free keto diet during this time.
- Consume only warm or room-temperature foods and drinks, avoiding cold or raw items for seven days.
- Consider trying longer fasts, starting gradually.
- Begin by delaying breakfast by an hour or two, and extend the fast as you're comfortable.
- Iron-rich foods (grass-fed beef, lentils, spinach) + vitamin C for absorption. Magnesium for cramp relief.

Exercise:

- Low-impact cardio
- Yoga & stretching
- Bodyweight exercises or light weight
- Lifting (5 lbs.)
- Pilates

Mantra:

"Today, I will give myself space to grow."

PHASE 2—Follicular: Days 7-11

Top Tips:

- Leave a mark on this world, show it your legacy.
- Focus on outcompeting yourself, not others, during this time.
- Embrace structure and discipline.
- Visualization and focus exercises—your brain is primed for planning.

Diet:

- Continue focusing on high protein and healthy fats.
- Increase your variety of vegetables—aim to "eat the rainbow" (Skittles don't count!)
- Add high-fat nuts and seeds, such as Brazil nuts, cashews, pumpkin seeds, and flax seeds.
- Consider trying a 24-hour fast if you're ready.
- Drink at least half your body weight in ounces of water to support your body.

- Liver-supportive foods (beets, dandelion greens, crucifers) to metabolize rising estrogen.

Exercise:

- Lift heavier weights (about 15 lbs. or what you feel comfortable with).
- HIIT—High Intensity Interval Training
- REHIT—Reduced Exertion High Intensity Training
- SIT—Sprint Interval Training

Mantra:
"Today is my opportunity to build the tomorrow I want."

PHASE 3—Ovulation: Days 12-15

Top Tips:

- Focus on achieving your goals.
- Manifest your dreams.
- Take advantage of your energy & drive.
- Social connections are important as they release oxytocin, which can amplify confidence and calm.

Diet:

- Incorporate raw and cold foods during this phase.
- Increase complex carbohydrates (not simple sugars).
- Focus on foods rich in selenium and vitamin E to support liver detox.
- Fasting is still beneficial, but keep fasts shorter—no longer than 17 hours.

- Zinc (pumpkin seeds, oysters) for egg quality and hormone balance. Selenium-rich foods (Brazil nuts) to support thyroid and estrogen metabolism.

Exercise:

- Lift heavier weights (about 20 lbs. or what you feel comfortable with).
- HIIT—High Intensity Interval Training
- REHIT—Reduced Exertion High Intensity Training
- SIT—Sprint Interval Training

Mantra:

"My energy is my life-source. She is a source of inspiration and action."

PHASE 4—Luteal: Days 16-28

Top Tips:

- Self-reflect by journaling or meditating.
- Mindful movement and journaling to lower PMS-related mood swings.
- Listen to your intuition.
- Look inward and listen to your body.
- Keep the bedroom cooler and avoid caffeine after midday to offset the drop in progesterone.

Diet:

- Lower your carb intake during the luteal phase.
- Be mindful of sugar cravings; drink water first to combat dehydration-related cravings.

- You can fast in the early days, but stop fasting by Day 20.
- Prioritize at least 30g of protein per meal.
- Aim to eat between 8 a.m. and 5 p.m.
- Focus on plenty of vegetables, lean meats, and wild-caught seafood.
- Vitamin B6 (chicken, salmon, bananas) to boost progesterone and ease PMS.

Exercise:

- Phase out high-intensity training
- Low-impact cardio
- Pilates
- Yoga/Stretching
- Bodyweight exercises or light weight
- Lifting (5 lbs.)

Mantra:

"I have the power to protect and renew my energy."

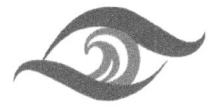

Hormone Disruptors: The Hidden Saboteurs in Your Daily Life

Let's talk about something that affects every single one of us, whether we realize it or not: hormone disruptors. Your endocrine system is a beautifully complex network made up of hormone-producing glands and receptors. This system helps regulate some of the body's most vital functions:

- Growth and development
- Metabolism and weight regulation
- Reproductive health
- Mood and brain function

But there's a problem, and it's everywhere.

What Are Endocrine Disruptors?

Endocrine disruptors are chemicals that interfere with your hormone balance. They either mimic your body's natural hormones or block them from doing their job. Because hormones work like keys fitting into very specific locks (your receptors), when a disruptor gets in there instead, it throws the entire system off. Unfortunately, these disruptors are all around us in places you may not even think about:

- Plastic bottles and containers
- Canned food linings
- Cleaning supplies
- Personal care products (yes, even "natural" ones)
- Flame-retardant materials (like furniture or pajamas)
- Nonorganic produce and conventional meat
- Toys, receipts, air fresheners, and more

We breathe them, eat them, apply them to our skin, and even absorb them through touch. And while we can't control everything, there's so much we can do once we know where to look.

You may be one of those people who says, "I'm fine, I'm not sensitive, and none of these things affect me in any way," but they do in one way or another. These chemicals are not harmless; they've been linked to:

- Stubborn belly fat (yes, they mess with metabolism and make fat loss way harder)
- Cognitive issues (including ADHD and memory problems)
- Immune dysfunction
- Infertility and menstrual issues
- Thyroid disruption
- Developmental delays in children
- Diabetes and metabolic disorders
- Certain hormone-related cancers

This isn't fearmongering, this is science. And the good news is that once you know, you can start reducing your exposure right away.

Endocrine Disruptors

Endocrine disruptor	Description	Possible sources
Bisphenol A (BPA)	A chemical used to produce hard plastic, such as polycarbonate	Canned beverages Canned food liners Dental sealants Kids toys Medical equipment Microwaveable food products Plastic food storage containers Plastic tableware Reusable water bottles Thermal paper receipts
Dioxins	Chemicals that have chlorine atoms as part of their structure are commonly emitted during fuel-burning processes, and can be found in food, water, soil, and air	Air during iron and steel production Air during the combustion of coal, oil, or wood Contaminated drinking water Dairy products Electrical power generation Fish and shellfish Meat Tobacco

Fragrances	Chemicals that emit volatile organic compounds (VOCs), such as limonene	Air fresheners Cleaning products Hand sanitizers Laundry supplies Personal care products Soaps
Parabens	Chemicals that are used as preservatives	Cosmetics Food products Personal care products Pharmaceuticals products
Perfluorinated chemicals (PFCs)	A class of chemicals that contribute to greenhouse gas emissions	Groundwater Firefighting foams Industrial products Microwave popcorn Non-stick cookware Paper Soil Textile coatings Waterproof clothing
Phthalates	A group of chemicals used to make plastics flexible	Detergents Diapers Food packaging Kids toys Personal care products (e.g., cosmetics, nail polish, shampoo) Sanitary napkins Vinyl flooring

Polybrominated diphenyl ethers (PBDE)	A chemical that's used as a flame retardant	Adhesives and sealants Appliances Automobile materials Carpet underlay Building materials Electrical equipment Furniture foam Mattresses Rubber products
Polychlorinated biphenyls (PCB)	Chemicals that break down slowly are traditionally found in industrial materials and are used to manufacture coolants or lubricants for electrical equipment such as capacitors and transformers	Adhesives and tapes Caulking Electrical equipment Fiberglass Fluorescent light ballasts Foam Oil-based paint Inks Plastics Sealants
Triclosan	A chemical with antimicrobial and antifungal activity	Liquid body washes Hand sanitizer Household products Mouthwash Surgical soaps Toothpaste

Xenoestrogens	Chemicals that may mimic estrogen in the body and interfere with the hormone's intended actions	Coolants
		Food preservatives
		Personal care products
		Pesticides
		Pharmaceuticals
		Plasticidants
		UV filters

Tips to Reduce Exposure

- Avoid scented products such as candles, perfumes, and air fresheners.
- Avoid using pesticides in the garden.
- Buy organic food when possible, and peel your fruits and vegetables.
- Choose personal care and cleaning products that don't contain toxic chemicals.
- Invest in a reusable glass or metal water bottle.
- Never reheat food in plastic containers.
- Opt for fresh foods instead of canned or microwavable meals.
- Replace your nonstick pots and pans if they become damaged.
- Store food and beverages in glass containers instead of plastic.
- Wash your vegetables and fruit before eating them.
- Use an app to help you evaluate ingredients for safety.

Helpful Apps to Detox Your Life

These free apps can help you make safer, healthier choices by scanning products and providing instant information about ingredients, toxins, and overall health impact. Use them while shopping or at home to detox your body and environment with confidence.

Detox Me Created by Silent Spring Institute, this app offers easy, science-based tips to reduce exposure to harmful chemicals in your everyday life.

→ Great for beginners who want step-by-step lifestyle detox guidance.

EWG's Healthy Living App From the Environmental Working Group, this app lets you scan food, cosmetics, and household products. It rates them based on toxicity and health concerns, using clean, transparent science.

→ Trusted by wellness professionals for ingredient safety checks.

Think Dirty Scan personal care and beauty products to find out what's really inside them. It breaks down ingredient toxicity and offers cleaner alternatives.

→ Especially helpful for makeup, shampoo, and skincare swaps.

Yuka Scan food and cosmetics to receive an easy-to-understand health score out of 100. Yuka flags harmful additives, colorants, and preservatives and recommends healthier options.

→ User-friendly with a clear visual scoring system.

Clean Living Swaps & Essentials

I've created an Amazon List with all of my favorite alternative products for your home, body, and kitchen. You can access it here:

https://amzn.to/45YMqFZ

You can also join our membership program, where you will receive up-to-date information about toxins and chemicals, new products, and so much more.

But if you're looking elsewhere, here are some easy, effective swaps to start detoxing your lifestyle:

Cookware

Switch out your non-stick pans for safer, non-toxic options like:

- Cast Iron—naturally nonstick once seasoned and adds iron to your food!
- Caraway—beautiful, nontoxic ceramic-coated cookware
- Our Place—multifunctional, aesthetically pleasing, and toxin-free

Ditch the Perfume

Fragrance = hidden chemicals. Instead, use essential oils like lavender, citrus, or sandalwood. They're therapeutic, customizable, and way healthier for your hormones.

Skin Moisturizer: Extra Virgin Olive Oil

Olive oil is an amazing, cheap, and effective alternative to chemical-laden lotions. It is hydrating, healing, and anti-inflammatory, great for diaper rashes, sunburns, bug bites, and more. Just don't use it on your face, it's too heavy and can clog pores.

Why use olive oil over coconut oil? Coconut oil molecules are too large to penetrate the skin effectively, so they tend to just sit on the surface, making it oily, messy, and easily transferred to clothes and sheets. Olive oil, on the other hand, absorbs much better.

Use companies like Counter, ASEA, DIME Beauty, The Honest Company, and Babz for all your makeup, skincare, and bodycare needs. These brands are leading the way in clean beauty by prioritizing nontoxic, cruelty-free ingredients, sustainable packaging, and transparent formulations that are safe for both your skin and the planet.

Whether you're looking for everyday essentials or elevated beauty rituals, clean beauty ensures you're not compromising your health in the name of self-care. Choosing clean means embracing products that nourish your skin from the outside in, without the harmful chemicals, endocrine disruptors, or synthetic fragrances found in conventional beauty.

Water Filtration Clean water is one of the most important health investments you can make.

- Berkey Filter—my top pick! Removes hormones, pharmaceuticals (like antidepressants), MTBE, heavy metals, and other contaminants while keeping in beneficial minerals.
- Reverse Osmosis—works well if you choose a system that:
  - Removes MTBE
  - Replenishes the minerals stripped from the water.

- Brita or fridge filters? Not enough. These don't remove the serious stuff.
- Whole House Solution: LifeSource is a great system if you want every faucet, shower, and tap in your home to be clean and toxin-free.

Fruit + Veggie Cleaning

We use an ozone bubbler to wash all our fruits and vegetables. It is affordable, powerful at removing pesticides, bacteria, and super easy to use.

Pro Tip: Dry your produce really well before storing it in the fridge, otherwise it wilts much faster!

Here is what I want you to understand.

We are what we …

- Eat
- Drink
- Breathe
- Touch
- … and what we can't eliminate

Here are some terms that I want you to know:

Body burden—the quantity of one exogenous substance (e.g., heavy metals, preservatives in cosmetics, BPA, phthalates, Red 40, Yellow 5, forever chemicals, xenobiotics, or any other chemical) or its metabolites that accumulate in an individual.

Total toxic load—the total body burden of exogenous chemicals, heavy metals, and toxic endogenous compounds.

Here is why this is important: each chemical is a burden on the body, but all of them combined become a toxic load. You might choose to wear chemical-filled makeup, put chemical-filled creams on your body, choose chemical nail polish, color your hair, eat nonorganic foods, and cook with nonstick pans.

Then you head out for a workout in your best-looking but mostly plastic athletic wear. As you sweat, your pores open wide, creating the perfect gateway for all those chemicals in the fabric to be absorbed straight into your skin at maximum capacity. Individually, they might not seem that harmful, but each adds a toxic burden to your body.

Do all of these constantly, add to that the toxins we breathe in the air, the water we shower in, and the steam particles we breathe in from the hot water, and it creates a toxic load on our bodies.

At some point, the toxic overload becomes too much, and the next toxin will be "the straw that breaks the camel's back": your body will give up, and disease will occur.

We even have equations to figure this out.

$$\text{Disease risk from toxic substances} = \text{Toxic potency} \times \text{cumulative exposure} \times \text{susceptibility}$$

There was a report published by Physicians for Social Responsibility, the American Nurses Association, and Health Care Without Harm on Hazardous Chemicals in Health Care. The repost showed that each nurse participant had at least 24 individual chemicals present in their body, four of which are on the Environmental Protection Agency's list of priority chemicals for regulation.[9]

My point here is that if we can't even look after our doctors and nurses in the hospitals where they work, how do *we* expect to be looked after? If getting your nails done is important to you, then try nontoxic nail polish or do it because it makes you feel amazing inside and out.

But then choose organic, grass-fed, or pasture-raised foods whenever possible, or make sure you are wearing 100% organic cotton underwear and other clothing, so that you decrease the toxic load on your body.

By the way, the top six chemicals found in doctors and nurses are:

- Bisphenol A (BPA)
- Mercury
- Perfluorinated compounds
- Phthalates
- Polybrominated diphenyl ethers
- Triclosan

---

[9] "The Risky Business of Nursing - Page 5," Medscape, January 14, 2014, https://www.medscape.com/viewarticle/818437_5?utm_source=chatgpt.com.

If you are one of those very sensitive individuals who, at this point, can't go outside because one sniff of a fragrance from a person that is walking on the other side of the street causes you to sneeze, break out in hives, or get a headache, there is a reason. You may have an increased or ongoing exposure to toxins.

You could be deficient in key nutrients like B vitamins, antioxidants, magnesium, or selenium. Your diet might be high in refined foods or low in clean protein. You may have intestinal dysbiosis, which means an imbalance in your gut bacteria. You may have genetic mutations that affect phase I and phase II of your detoxification pathways. Or you may even be carrying unresolved emotional trauma or experiencing chronic stress.

Each year, thousands of new chemicals are introduced into the global market, and estimates suggest that over 2,000 new substances are added annually (EVERY DAMN YEAR). While regulatory agencies like the EPA or ECHA require some level of safety testing, only a small fraction are thoroughly evaluated for long-term human health effects, especially in real-world, low-dose exposures.

What is even more concerning is that the vast majority of chemicals are tested in isolation only, not in the combinations we're routinely exposed to through food, air, water, and personal care products. Studies examining the cumulative or combined effects of multiple chemicals, often called the "cocktail effect," are rare and severely underfunded, even though there is a mountain of growing evidence that combined exposures can amplify toxicity or disrupt biological systems, such as hormones, immune function, or the gut microbiome.

Infertility, allergies, autoimmune diseases, cancers, and childhood diseases are all on the rise, but this regulatory gap leaves many chemicals on the market without a clear understanding of their impact on human health, especially over time and across generations.

At this point, we will always have toxins in our lives, but add the ones you really can't live without and try to decrease the rest as much as you can.

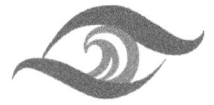

Your Only Limit Is You

Muscle Is the Organ of Longevity

Dr. Gabrielle Lyon points out that skeletal muscle is not merely for movement but functions as a vital endocrine organ. Healthy muscle mass enhances metabolism, regulates blood sugar, supports immune function, and contributes to cognitive health. Prioritizing muscle health can delay or prevent chronic diseases and improve overall quality of life as we age.

The four diseases that are killing most people are also preventable:

- Heart disease
- Cancer
- Neurodegenerative disease (like Alzheimer's)
- Type 2 diabetes and metabolic dysfunction

None of these diseases, especially Alzheimer's and dementia, begin in old age; they often start with poor metabolic health, inflammation, and inactivity. So exercise, fasting, sleep hygiene, blood sugar control, and stress reduction are so important. No drug or intervention comes close to the benefit of exercise. It reduces risk for all four of the above diseases.

Here are just some of the benefits of exercise:

1. **Cognitive protection**
    - Physical activity increases brain-derived neurotrophic factor (BDNF). Think of it as brain fertilizer.
    - Reduces risk of Alzheimer's and vascular dementia
    - Increases blood flow and improves executive function, memory, and mood

2. **Cardiovascular health**
    - VO2 max (your maximum oxygen uptake) is one of the strongest predictors of all-cause mortality.
    - Exercise improves insulin sensitivity, lowers blood pressure, balances lipids, and reduces inflammation, all of which protect the heart and arteries.

3. **Muscle mass = life insurance**
    - Sarcopenia (age-related muscle loss) is a major cause of frailty, falls, and loss of independence.
    - Maintaining lean muscle helps with:
        - Blood sugar control
        - Metabolic flexibility
        - Joint and bone health
        - Stability and injury prevention

The goal is to be able to perform the functional physical tasks you want to be able to do at age 100.

For example:

- Pick up your grandkids
- Climb stairs without help
- Carry groceries
- Get up off the floor without assistance

To achieve this, you have to train for it today. Your future self depends on the foundation you build in your 40s, 50s, and 60s. We mentioned earlier that muscle strengthening and stretching are equally important.

I am not sure how many of you are aware of it, but most of the health and fitness studies and therefore the wearables that we have to date are based on men, usually 5 ft. 10 inches, white, aged between 25-35, weighing around 165 lbs. Women are comparing themselves to what their wearables are telling them, but the wearables are based on men . . . this just blows my mind!

Dr. Stacy Sims, a performance physiologist specializing in female health, challenges the popular notion that "Zone 2" cardio (around 60–70% of max heart rate) is universally optimal. She explains that women naturally have a higher density of slow-twitch muscle fibers, more mitochondria, and better oxidative metabolism than men, so the mitochondrial benefits of prolonged, moderate-intensity exercise are less pronounced in women.

Instead, she recommends that women prioritize high-intensity interval training (HIIT—45-50 seconds) and sprint interval training (SIT), short bursts of intense work (15-20 seconds) with rest, about two to four times per week to effectively enhance mitochondrial function, insulin sensitivity, visceral fat loss, and brain health.[10]

Zone 2 doesn't have to be eliminated; it's great for active recovery, but should be balanced with higher-intensity sessions, especially as women navigate midlife transitions and hormone changes. This approach not only aligns with female physiology but also supports optimal metabolic, skeletal, and cognitive health. Thank god for doctors like Dr. Stacy Sims, Dr. Gabrielle Lyon, and many more, who are pointing out how different men and women are (as if it wasn't obvious already).

Zone 2 cardio (endurance)

- Low-intensity, long-duration (think fast walking, biking, easy jogging), you can breathe through your nose and hold a conversation
- Improves mitochondrial function, fat metabolism, and cardiovascular health
- Aim for 3–5 hours per week

---

[10] Stacy T. Sims, *Roar: How to Match Your Food and Fitness to Your Unique Female Physiology for Optimum Performance, Great Health, and a Strong, Lean Body for Life* (Emmaus, PA: Rodale Books, 2016).

VO2 max/high-intensity training

- Short bursts of all-out effort (e.g., sprints, HIIT)
- Increases cardiovascular reserve and capacity
- Linked to longer life and better stress resilience
- 2-3 sessions/week is often enough (20-minute sessions are perfect)

Strength training

- Builds muscle mass, supports metabolism, and strengthens bones
- Helps prevent falls, fractures, and functional decline
- At least 2–3 full-body resistance sessions per week

Stability & mobility

- Often overlooked but critical as we age
- Focus on balance, core strength, joint mobility, and posture
- Prevents injury and helps maintain independence

Functional Health Tests

Here's a functional strength benchmark chart by age group for both men and women. These are general targets based on fitness research, functional medicine guidelines, and longevity studies. They can help you assess biological vs. chronological aging and track resilience over time.

Men's Functional Strength Benchmarks by Age
(General guidelines for healthy, injury-free individuals)

Test	Color	Age 20–39	Age 40–59	Age 60+
Dead Hang (Grip Strength)	Green	90 sec	60 sec	45 sec
	Yellow	72–89 sec	48–59 sec	36 44 sec
	Red	<72 sec	<48 sec	<36 sec

Why It Matters: Grip strength is a longevity predictor and reflects nervous system health.

Push-Ups (Upper Body)	Green	25–35	20–30	'10–20
	Yellow	20–24	16–19	'8–9
	Red	<20	<16	<8

Why It Matters: Measures upper body and core strength; important for posture and mobility.

Wall Sit (Lower Body)	Green	90 sec	60 sec	45 sec
	Yellow	72–89 sec	48–59 sec	36–44 sec
	Red	<72 sec	<48 sec	<36 sec

Why It Matters: Assesses quad/glute endurance and knee stability.

Sit-to-Stand (1 min)	Green	20–25	15–20	'12–15
	Yellow	16–19	'12–14	'10–11
	Red	<16	<12	<10

Why It Matters: Strong predictor of long-term independence and leg power.

Plank Hold (Core)	Green	2–3 min	60–120 sec	60–90 sec
	Yellow	96–119 sec	48–59 sec	48–59 sec
	Red	<96 sec	<48 sec	<48 sec

Why It Matters: Core strength = spinal support, injury prevention, metabolic regulation.

Single-Leg Balance	Green	30–60 sec	30 sec	15–20 sec
	Yellow	24–29 sec	24–29 sec	12–14 sec
	Red	<24 sec	<24 sec	<12 sec

Why It Matters: Critical for neurological health and fall prevention.

Women's Functional Strength Benchmarks by Age
(General guidelines for healthy, injury-free individuals)

Test		Age 20–39	Age 40–59	Age 60+
Dead Hang (Grip Strength)	Green	60 sec	45 sec	30 sec
	Yellow	48–59 sec	36–44 sec	24–29 sec
	Red	<48 sec	<36 sec	<24 sec

Why It Matters: Grip strength is a longevity predictor and reflects nervous system health.

Push-Ups (Upper Body)	Green	15–20	10–15	5–10
	Yellow	12–14	8–9	4
	Red	'12	'8	<4

Why It Matters: Measures upper body and core strength; important for posture and mobility.

Wall Sit (Lower Body)	Green	>90 sec	>60 sec	>45 sec
	Yellow	72–89 sec	48–59 sec	36–44 sec
	Red	<72 sec	<48 sec	<36 sec

Why It Matters: Assesses quad/glute endurance and knee stability.

Sit-to-Stand (1 min)	Green	20–25	15–20	12–15
	Yellow	16–19	12–14	10–11
	Red	<16	<12	<10

Why It Matters: Strong predictor of long-term independence and leg power.

Plank Hold (Core)	Green	>120 sec	90 sec	45–60 sec
	Yellow	96–119 sec	72–89 sec	36–44 sec
	Red	<96 sec	<72 sec	<36 sec

Why It Matters: Core strength = spinal support, injury prevention, metabolic regulation.

Single-Leg Balance	Green	30 60 sec	30 sec	15 20 sec
	Yellow	24 29 sec	24 29 sec	12 14 sec
	Red	<24 sec	<24 sec	<12 sec

Why It Matters: Critical for neurological health and fall prevention.

How to Use This Chart

- Green Zone = You're hitting or exceeding your target = biologically resilient
- Yellow Zone = Slightly below target = room for improvement
- Red Zone = Significantly below = time to re-evaluate lifestyle, mobility, and training

Note: Your connective tissue, especially fascia, is like your body's built-in Wi-Fi system. It's not just holding everything together; it's constantly sending messages between your muscles, nerves, and brain.

This web of tissue senses movement, tension, and pressure, helping your body stay balanced, coordinated, and aware. It's also full of fluid and receptors that pass signals faster than nerves alone, making it a super-efficient communication system.

That's why stretching, breath work, or foam rolling can instantly make you feel calmer, looser, and more in tune with your body. Fascia is your body's secret messenger network, keeping everything connected, literally and energetically!

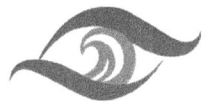

The Sleep Prescription

Let's Talk About Sleep

Sleep is essential, not optional. It's just as vital to your health as food and water. Chronic sleep deprivation is linked to serious health issues like heart disease, diabetes, obesity, and Alzheimer's.

Most adults need between seven and nine hours of sleep each night, and even losing just an hour or two can negatively impact their memory, immune system, metabolism, and mood.

There are two main types of sleep: REM (Rapid Eye Movement) and non-REM. Both are equally important. Non-REM sleep supports learning and memory consolidation, while REM sleep enhances creativity and emotional resilience.

During sleep, especially deep sleep, your brain cleans itself, literally. It activates what's called the glymphatic system, a waste-clearing process that flushes out toxins like beta-amyloid, which is associated with Alzheimer's disease. Interestingly, sleeping on your right side may help this process work more efficiently.

REM sleep also supports your emotional regulation. It helps your brain process the events and emotions of the day and lowers your reactivity to emotional stress the next day.

Without enough sleep, your problem-solving skills, attention span, and ability to regulate your emotions all suffer, often without you realizing how impaired you are.

One of the most shocking facts is that being awake for 20 hours straight affects your reflexes as much as being legally drunk. Drowsy driving is just as dangerous as drunk driving.

Sleep also plays a huge role in your immune system. Just one night of only four or five hours of sleep can reduce natural killer cell activity, your cancer-fighting immune cells, by up to 70%. That's how powerful sleep is. During sleep, the body also replenishes its energy storage, regenerates tissue, and produces proteins.

Of course, there are things that can sabotage sleep. Caffeine blocks adenosine, a sleep-promoting chemical, so it's best to avoid it in the afternoon or evening. Alcohol might help you fall asleep, but it disrupts your sleep architecture and suppresses REM sleep.

If you love your evening wine, that's okay, but try to reduce the number of nights you drink. Start by going from seven nights to five, then three. Your sleep will thank you.

Also, avoid screens before bed. The blue light emitted from phones, tablets, and TVs suppresses melatonin—the hormone that tells your body it's time to wind down. Try to unplug one to two hours before bedtime, or at the very least, keep devices away from your body while sleeping.

Sleep affects your systolic blood pressure, metabolism, and weight too. It disrupts the hormones ghrelin and leptin, which regulate hunger and fullness. That's why when you're sleep-deprived, you tend to crave more food and often the worst kind.

If you're someone who struggles with emotional eating, improving your sleep could help tremendously. Staying up late releases a shot of cortisol, which we know increases cell signaling to cytokines (molecules of inflammation). I know you heard a lot about the cytokine storm during COVID.

Circadian rhythms are biological processes linked to the cycles of the day. Many bodily functions vary according to these rhythms.

- Body temperature
- Pulse rate and blood pressure
- Reaction time and performance
- The production of melatonin, serotonin, and cortisol
- Intestinal activity

Your internal clock resets itself daily when it is exposed to sunlight. That's why sleeping in a dark, cold room is best for sleep, and then opening up those blinds first thing in the morning and getting a blast of full-spectrum light is so important.

Teenagers, by the way, need even more sleep than adults, about 8 to 10 hours per night. But with early school start times and packed schedules, most aren't getting anywhere close. This affects not just learning, but also mood and mental health. Honestly, we should be rethinking the entire school structure, changing the hours, improving the food, and redesigning how we teach.

While naps can be a helpful supplement, they're not a substitute for deep, restorative night sleep. Short naps of 20–30 minutes can boost alertness and productivity, but they don't replace the benefits of a full night's sleep.

And no, you can't "catch up" on sleep. That's a myth. Sleep debt adds up quickly, and it takes about 10 days of consistent, quality sleep to recover from just one night of poor sleep.

Side note: A newborn baby does not start producing melatonin until they are three months old, so be patient with the baby and yourself. If you have older kids who do not sleep, then do what you can whenever you can.

I have two kids who are now 5 and a quarter (as he likes to tell everyone) and 8, and they still wake me up once or twice most nights because they want a snuggle, are sick, had a nightmare, or want a foot, hand, or head massage (my kids are spoiled!).

You should look at why your child is not sleeping. Are they eating or drinking too late, have too much sugar in their diet, not eating enough, their room is either too cold or too hot, or too noisy or not noisy enough? Also, too much screen time before bed increases levels of dopamine and serotonin, which causes alertness and therefore disturbs sleep.

Whatever it may be, you may need to sage and Palo Santo (a natural cleansing herb) the room to get rid of bad energy. Try what you can and get rest when you can.

All I can tell you is that at some point it will all even out, and your children will start sleeping, but you stressing out even more that you have to sleep but are not sleeping because of the kids will cause you even more harm. Take a breath or 20, and try to fall back asleep!

Tips for Improving Sleep
Setting up Your Room

- Make your room as dark as possible by using blackout shades.
- Cover the LEDs on your electronics with black tape (or better yet, avoid having any electronics in your room).
- Switch lamps to brands that do not emit the blue light spectrum (e.g., lamps that change the spectrum of light according to the cycle of day or dim salt lamps).

Bed Quality

- Mattress made of organic cotton, wool, hemp, or natural rubber
- Oat, cherry, spelt, or buckwheat pillow
- Organic cotton or silk sheets
- Sleep naked—sometimes the rubber bands around your waist can cut off your lymphatic flow.
- Sleep without a pillow or use one that supports your neck well.
- Sleep with a pillow between your legs when sleeping on your side.
- The ideal sleep position is on your back or your right side.

Electromagnetic Pollution

- No electronics in your room.
- Turn off your Wi-Fi at night.
- Use grounding mats while you sleep and work at your computer.

- Walk barefoot during the day in grass or sand.
- Use EMF blockers.

Air Quality

- Ventilate your room during the day.
- Test for mold.
- Use plants to increase humidity, turn carbon dioxide into oxygen, and release negative ions.
- Use UV, HEPA, carbon filters, and an air ionizer.

Temperature

- Ideally 64-69F
- Prepare during the day to get better sleep at night.
- Spend time in the sunlight 20 minutes in the morning before 11 a.m. and 20 minutes in the evening after 4 p.m.
- Avoid sunglasses; they trick your brain into thinking it's night.
- Do 20-30 minutes of exercise daily—any type of exercise.
- Avoid stress as much as possible. I know it's hard, so counteract your stress with a nightly Epsom salt bath, a massage, sauna, breath work, or some light stretching.

Getting Ready for Bed

- Take nutrients that will help you sleep—magnesium citrate, tryptophan, reishi mushroom, l-theanine, and zinc, just to name a few.
- Avoid caffeine, alcohol, bacon, cheese, chocolate, sausage, potatoes, and tomatoes before bed if you are sensitive to them.

- Keep hydrated throughout the day.
- Keep your body temperature lower before bed, so no evening exercising.
- Take some breaths and meditate.
- Avoid blue light.
- Breathe through your nose (tape your mouth if you have to).

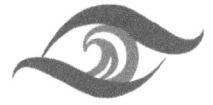

Pills with Purpose

Let's Talk About Supplements

I love supplements, and I believe they're necessary, especially because our soil here in the States is so incredibly depleted. We are not getting the same nutrients out of our food that we used to in the 40s and 50s, or even the same nutrients that other countries have in their foods. Have you ever tasted a tomato from Europe, New Zealand, or South America? If you haven't, you really need to. It will blow your mind about the amount of flavor a simple vegetable has!

But I also believe we're overdoing supplementation. The truth is, even if your digestion is functioning optimally, you're probably only absorbing 30 to 35 percent of the supplements you take by mouth. That's why IV vitamins can be so effective; they go directly into your bloodstream, offering nearly 100 percent absorption. However, IV therapy isn't always accessible and can be expensive.

The source and quality of your supplements matter just as much as what you're taking. Cheaper options from big box stores like Costco, Amazon, or CVS often contain low-quality ingredients, weak dosages, or poor formulations. Not to mention that Amazon sells counterfeit supplements that look almost exactly like the real thing. It's crazy and scary. You end up wasting money and not getting any of the promised benefits.

Practitioner-grade supplements, on the other hand, are made with higher standards in mind. They offer better bioavailability and are rigorously tested for purity and potency. I personally use and recommend Fullscript, a platform that carries only trusted, practitioner-grade brands. You can browse by category, read up on ingredients, and find what aligns with your needs:

> https://us.fullscript.com/plans/awakennow-awaken-now-guide

That said, always consult with your doctor before adding anything new to your supplement routine, especially if you're on medications. Safety first!

If you'd like to explore individual supplements in more depth and learn how they might support your unique goals, our membership program offers a space for continued learning, growth, and experimentation to find what works best for you.

You'll find extra resources, teaching videos, and inspiring challenges, all designed to help you build momentum toward your health goals and get back more than you put in.

While everything I've shared so far is true and important, this next section, in my opinion, is the most important. This is the cherry on top that can permanently transform your life for the better, or the straw that can break the camel's back, in which case you'll reread everything, start your daily prompts, and pick your damn self back up again!

If you change your diet, take supplements, and exercise, you will see improvement. You might even feel great, better than ever! But you will never feel truly whole until you master your mind.

With the right mindset, everything you implement will happen faster, more easily, and with greater long-term impact.

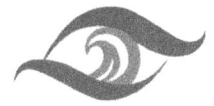

Spirit & Science: The Missing Link in Health

Let's Talk Spirituality and Mindset

Spirituality is your connection to something greater than yourself, whether that's nature, intuition, love, purpose, or a divine source. It's what grounds you, guides you through life's challenges, inspires personal growth, and brings a sense of peace.

Mindset refers to how you think, feel, and act in your daily life.

Are you the "glass half empty" type or the "glass half full" type?

Do you say things like, "This is just who I am," or do you think, "I can learn from this and adjust next time"?

This is the practice of monitoring your thoughts. You can't evolve, grow, or transform if you're constantly playing the game of life from within your blind spots.

We'll talk more about that in a moment. By the way, while you're learning to monitor your thoughts, don't get mad at yourself for slipping into old habits. Instead, celebrate the fact that you caught yourself! That's progress. Next time, you'll catch it sooner and kick that habit's ass.

To figure out where you stand, ask yourself these three questions:

- "Do I believe I can grow and change?"
- "Do I see challenges as threats or as opportunities?"
- "Do I trust myself to handle what life throws at me?"

Why Mindset Matters . . . Scientifically

Do you know what separates us from every other species on this planet?

It's the size and complexity of our frontal lobe in relation to the rest of the brain. The frontal lobe is the part of the brain responsible for:

- setting firm intentions
- making decisions
- regulating behavior
- accessing inspiration and higher thinking

Here's what happens:

1. We take in information from our environment.
2. We process that information.
3. We store it in our brain.
4. Then, we're able to make new choices and decisions that differ from those we've made in the past.

A Little Brain Science

The brain is made up of tiny nerve cells called neurons. These neurons have tiny branches that reach out and connect with other neurons to form what's called a neural net.

Every time they connect, that connection becomes a piece of a thought or a memory. Thoughts, feelings, and experiences are built into this network. They're all interconnected, and they all influence each other.

For example, if you associate love with pain, your brain doesn't know the difference between what it's remembering and what it's currently seeing in the environment because the same neural networks are firing.

Let's say you've been hurt by a past lover. Then one day, you're out at a coffee shop and you see a couple quietly sitting in the corner. Suddenly, your mind starts spinning about why they are not talking:

- "He probably did something to her."
- "She expects way too much from him."
- "He even looks like a narcissist."
- "I bet she just said …"

You're reliving that old pain, projecting it onto the world around you because those neurons wired with pain are firing again. Your past has become your lens, and all you actually saw was a couple sitting quietly.

Now, let's take something like menopause. You expect hot flashes, insomnia, weight gain, and aging because everyone talks about it that way. When you sit down with your girlfriends and the conversation turns into a group vent session, all that emotion, energy, and passion strengthen those thoughts and beliefs.

You start expecting hardship … and that's exactly what you experience. You've seen your mother, your sister, or your aunt struggle, so naturally, you assume you will too.

Remember when we talked about perceived stress, epigenetics, and how your thoughts write their story directly into your DNA? This is it. But here's the good news: you can use this same system for good.

Train Your Mind Like an Athlete Trains Their Body

Think of an Olympic athlete. They visualize their race every night before bed. The swimmer, runner, or basketball player doesn't just see the game; they feel it. Their muscles fire in the exact sequence as if it were real.

That's because the brain doesn't know the difference between imagination and reality when done with emotional intensity. If you imagine something, act as if it's already true, and feel the feelings as if it has happened, then the brain writes it as real.

Yes, this is the most "woo-woo" part of the book, I promise, but also … it's the fastest way to change your life.

"Nerve Cells That Fire Together, Wire Together"

If you practice something over and over again, your neurons develop long-term relationships.

But if you constantly get angry, stressed, or suffer daily, you're just reinforcing those neural networks. Here's the great news: You can stop those neurons from firing together just by interrupting the thought process.

This works the same as growing a muscle. You don't go to the gym once and expect abs. Rewiring your brain takes consistency. And the fastest way to get there? Celebrate your small victories.

I mean everything:

- You got a great parking spot? Celebrate.
- You watched an ant and guessed it would turn right—and it did? Celebrate.
- Someone bought your coffee? Celebrate.
- You caught yourself slipping into a bad habit? Celebrate.
- You didn't slip into a bad habit? Definitely celebrate.
- You had an amazing day, a magical date, a quiet bath? Yep, celebrate that too.

There's no win too small to honor, because every celebration changes your body chemistry and raises your vibration. Before you know it, you're on a whole new path, one that's been waiting for you, that you deserve, and that you're destined for.

You have a part of your brain called the hypothalamus, and it's like a chemical factory. It produces peptides, which are small chains of amino acids that match the emotions you experience.

There are peptides for anger, joy, sadness, lust, victimhood, and, honestly, anything and everything you can think of. Once produced, these peptides enter your bloodstream and attach to cells. The more frequently you experience a particular emotion, the more those peptides bombard your cells.

So what happens when your body constantly receives peptides for stress, anger, or guilt? When your cells divide, the daughter cells create more receptor sites for those specific emotional peptides and fewer for things like vitamins, minerals, nutrients, fluid exchange, or toxin release.

Over time, those peptides embed themselves into protein structures, and when protein production goes offtrack, we age. Let's break it down:

- Elastin in your skin? A protein.
- Digestive enzymes? Proteins.
- Synovial fluid in your joints? Proteins.
- Bone matrix? Protein-based.

All of these proteins can become stiff, brittle, or ineffective when they are emotionally imprinted the wrong way. So yes, it does matter what you eat, how you sleep, and how much you exercise, but if your cells no longer have the proper receptors to absorb health, then you're fighting an uphill battle.

This is where biochemistry meets behavior. When your cellular environment is shaped by repeated emotional patterns, those patterns start to dictate how your body functions, sometimes so strongly that they become addictive.

Naturally, your next question is going to be, "What is addiction?" Addiction is when you cannot control your emotional state. You become chemically attached to familiar feelings, whether they serve you or not. The emotions you cycle through in a 24-hour period reflect your internal thought patterns. And your thoughts either weaken or strengthen you. It's your choice.

Spirituality, in all its beautiful and personal forms—whether it's prayer, meditation, time in nature, or conversations about purpose—has the power to keep you youthful, calm, and resilient. And now, let's introduce a game-changing idea.

Let's Talk Vibrations & Frequencies

Our emotional state literally affects the frequency at which we vibrate. According to David Hawkins' book *Letting Go* (I highly recommend it!), here's how it breaks down:

- Shame vibrates at 20 Hz (the lowest)
- Guilt, fear, anger—still low, but higher than shame
- Courage is 200 Hz—this is where positive change begins
- Love, joy, peace—even higher
- Enlightenment—1000 Hz, the highest possible state

You don't want to get stuck in low emotions. Yes, we all feel them, and that's completely okay. The key is to move through them, not live in them.

Remember one of the universal laws: "Like attracts like." The more anger, guilt, stress, shame, or jealousy you carry, the more the universe will respond by sending you people and situations that trigger those same emotions. It has to. That's how the law works.

Until you consciously choose to let go and see the situation—or the person—differently, nothing changes. But the moment you shift your perception, you shift your frequency. And that's when life starts responding differently too.

And guess what? If you have the courage to take responsibility, shift your thoughts, and elevate your emotions, you can create anything. You can bend reality, manifest your dream life, and age backward from the inside out.

Map of Consciousness
Developed by David R. Hawkins

Name of Level	Energetic Log	Predominant Emotional State	View of Life	God-view	Process
Enlightenment	700-1000	Ineffable	Is	Self	Pure Consciousness
Peace	600	Bliss	Perfect	All-Being	Illumination
Joy	540	Serenity	Complete	One	Transfiguration
Love	500	Reverence	Benign	Loving	Revelation
Reason	400	Understanding	Meaningful	Wise	Abstraction
Acceptance	350	Forgiveness	Harmonious	Merciful	Transcendence
Willingness	310	Optimism	Hopeful	Inspiring	Intention
Neutrality	250	Trust	Satisfactory	Enabling	Release
Courage	200	Affirmation	Feasible	Permitting	Empowerment
Pride	175	Scorn	Demanding	Indifferent	Inflation
Anger	150	Hate	Antagonistic	Vengeful	Aggression
Desire	125	Craving	Disappointing	Denying	Enslavement
Fear	100	Anxiety	Frightening	Punitive	Withdrawal
Grief	75	Regret	Tragic	Disdainful	Despondency
Apathy	50	Despair	Hopeless	Condemning	Abdication
Guilt	30	Blame	Evil	Vindictive	Destruction
Shame	20	Humiliation	Miserable	Despising	Elimination

Spiritual Paradigm: Enlightenment–Love
Reason & Integrity: Reason–Courage
Survival Paradigm: Pride–Shame

Levels of Consciousness

I've recently been diving into the spiritual teachings of Kabbalah, and I have to say, it's been profoundly eye-opening. Kabbalah teaches that before we come to Earth, our souls choose everything: the people we'll meet, the relationships we'll have, and even the challenges we'll face. Why? So that our soul can grow and evolve.

You've probably met someone who just seems wise beyond their years, and you've thought, "Wow, they're an old soul." That's because they are. They've lived many lives, learned their lessons, and chosen growth over stagnation.

Here's the powerful part: you can do the same. What if your soul did invite that challenge? Let's say someone cuts you off in traffic. You slam on your brakes, honk your horn, and fume about it for the rest of the day, telling anyone who'll listen. Now, maybe you're justified.

But here's a little soul test. What if your soul invited that experience? What if that frustrating moment wasn't about the other driver, but about your reaction? What if your anger is the lesson?

The next time something triggers you, take a breath and try saying, "What a pleasure." Yes, seriously, "What a pleasure." Thank the moment for showing up so your soul can stretch, grow, and evolve, because if you do and you learn the lesson, you won't need to repeat it. You'll vibrate at a higher level, and life will begin to reflect that back to you.

This doesn't mean life gets easier; it means YOU get stronger. Choosing to evolve doesn't mean you'll stop facing challenges. But the quality of those challenges will grow with you. They'll feel less like obstacles and more like opportunities. Instead of staying stuck in guilt, shame, or anger, you'll start moving through those emotions faster and with more grace.

Some days you'll nail it.

Some days you'll fall flat on your face.

And other days you'll land somewhere in the messy middle. That's okay, just remember, every time you catch yourself and choose growth, you win. Celebrate every one of those moments.

And just so you know, even though I practice this with my patients and live it as best I can, I still mess up. Constantly. I still catch myself stuck in low emotions or reacting instead of responding.

But I keep showing up. I keep choosing evolution. Because let's be real, how sad is it to see someone still stuck in the same emotional loops years later? Living in anger or shame and calling it "just how I am"?

That's not living. That's surviving, and I can tell you from personal experience that being a survivor of life in general doesn't get you anywhere special, and even if you eventually get something "special" in one part of your life, it doesn't mean that the rest of your life is fulfilled. Something will always be missing, and whatever you do achieve will be achieved with great difficulty, stress, and strain.

I don't want to just survive, I want to grow. I want to evolve. And I want that for you too.

If this message resonates with you, and you're curious to dive deeper into Kabbalah, I highly recommend David

Ghiyam's course, www.davidghiyam.com, or you can do any of the fundamental courses at onehouse.kabbalah.com. It's interesting, challenging in just the right way, fun, and super affordable!

Let's not forget, chronic stress is aging you. And spirituality, whatever that may look like for you, is the antidote! Whether it's prayer, meditation, time in nature, journaling, or simply deep, meaningful conversations, connecting to something greater than yourself calms the nervous system, lowers inflammation, boosts immunity, and literally helps you age more slowly.

A bonus is that it often comes with a soul tribe: a meditation group, a book club, a circle of curious seekers, a community that heals. You feel more alive, more joyful, and yep, you glow from the inside out.

Think of spirituality as the ultimate stress detox. Let's be honest, stress is one of the biggest culprits behind premature aging. But when you make time to slow down, breathe deeply, and tap into gratitude or mindfulness, your whole system relaxes. That peace ripples through your body, lowering inflammation, boosting immunity, and giving your nervous system a much-needed vacation.

One more important thing that I want you to stay aware of. As you are consciously changing, growing, and evolving, the people who are around you in all aspects of your life—work, family, and friends—may start to slowly disappear from your life, no matter how much you love them and think you can't live without them.

Not because you will have a falling out or because something bad will happen, but simply because your vibrations and frequencies will start to rise the more you work on yourself. If the people around you choose not to work on themselves, to grow and evolve, that is okay. You can't make anyone change who is not ready for change, but make sure that you don't stop working on yourself just because your friends are not working on themselves.

Sometimes, evolution may get lonely; it may feel like you are changing and want to talk about different things or have different experiences than everyone else around you, as if you are moving forward, and everyone else is still at the starting line.

If you ever feel that way, where you are looking around and nothing feels comfortable, maybe you even have a higher level of unexplained anxiety, and you don't see anyone that you connect with, JUST KEEP GOING FORWARD.

You will eventually catch up with the new group of people who are meant to enter your life, those who are on the same frequency as you, with similar goals, and you will fit in so easily, as if you have known them forever!

The worst thing you can do is allow the fear of loneliness and discomfort to take over, causing you to stop growing and evolving and go right back to your comfort zone, your old life, your old friends, your old self—especially when your soul is itching for growth and evolution. You must have seen this sketch before; it explains it perfectly!

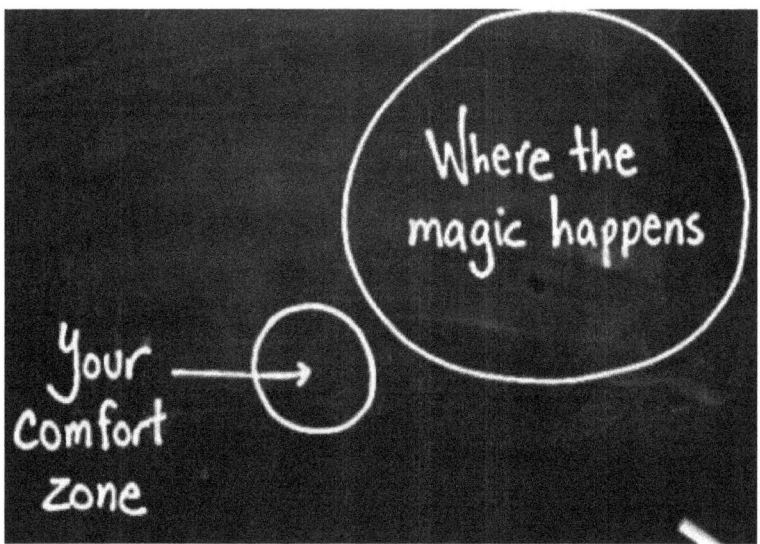

The 5 Whys

I want to introduce you to the "5 Whys" technique. This is for the times when you really get stuck in the lower emotional frequencies! Originally, this technique was developed by Sakichi Toyoda and popularized within Toyota's Lean Manufacturing system as a problem-solving method where you ask "Why?" five times to get to the root cause of an issue.

While it began in engineering and operations, it has been adapted by many self-help and personal development authors. The why is not there to help you justify why you did or said something that maybe could have been phrased better! Rather, the purpose is to dig deeper into yourself to see what you are lacking that caused the reaction you had. It is about honest, compassionate digging, getting to the emotional root so you can finally heal it. Here are a few examples for you to think about.

Problem:

"Why do I always pick bad partners?"
The 5 Whys:

1. Why do I always pick bad partners?
   → Because I'm attracted to certain traits that end up being toxic.

2. Why am I attracted to traits that end up being toxic?
   → Because those traits feel familiar or exciting at first.

3. Why do familiar or exciting traits draw me in, even when they're unhealthy?
   → Because they remind me of dynamics I experienced growing up or in early relationships.

4. Why do I subconsciously repeat those early dynamics?
   → Because part of me is trying to "fix" or "redeem" a past pain through present choices.

5. Why do I feel the need to fix or redeem the past through my relationships?
   → Because I haven't fully healed from those early wounds or learned to believe I deserve something healthier.

Problem:

"Why can't I lose weight or reach my health goals?"

The 5 Whys:

1. Why can't I lose weight or reach my health goals?
   → Because I struggle to stay consistent with healthy habits.

2. Why do I struggle to stay consistent with healthy habits?

→ Because I often feel overwhelmed or stressed and fall back into comfort behaviors like emotional eating or skipping workouts.

3. Why do I turn to emotional eating or skip workouts when I'm overwhelmed or stressed?

    → Because food and rest feel like immediate relief, and I don't have other go-to tools to self-regulate.

4. Why don't I have healthier tools to manage stress or emotional discomfort?

    → Because I was never taught how to process emotions in a healthy way, I learned to numb or avoid them.

5. Why haven't I learned to process emotions or build better coping strategies yet?

    → Because I've been focusing on fixing symptoms (diet/workout) instead of addressing the deeper emotional and mindset patterns driving my behavior.

Problem: "Why do I have so much anxiety?"

The 5 Whys:

1. Why do I have so much anxiety?

    → Because I often feel like things are out of my control and something bad might happen.

2. Why do I feel like things are out of my control?

    → Because I'm constantly thinking about worst-case scenarios and trying to plan for every possible outcome.

3. Why am I always thinking about worst-case scenarios?

   → Because I feel safer when I'm prepared. It's my way of trying to prevent pain, failure, or disappointment.

4. Why do I feel the need to prevent pain or failure so strongly?

   → Because in the past, I experienced situations where I felt blindsided, helpless, or unsafe, and I never fully processed or healed from that.

5. Why haven't I healed from those past experiences?

   → Because I've been focused on surviving, staying busy, or avoiding the discomfort rather than creating space to feel, process, and release what's still stuck.

Right now, every challenge you're facing is a message.

Every emotion is feedback.

Every person, especially the difficult ones, is a teacher.

So, the next time life tests you and you get stuck in a lower-frequency emotion, experiencing obsessive-compulsive thoughts and repetitive thoughts, pause, take a breath, and whisper, "What a pleasure."

Then choose your next step with intention, because your soul is asking for growth; it didn't come here to stay stuck. It came here to grow.

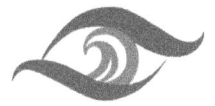

And Here We Are ... The End (Or the Beginning)

You made it, not just to the end of this book, but to the beginning of something amazing. The fact that you picked up this book and chose to read through it already says so much about who you are. I hope you learned something new, something that made you pause and reflect, and something that sparks real change.

Remember, every single thing you do—what you eat, how you move, how you sleep, and how you manage stress—affects your epigenetics. That may sound a little intimidating at first, and honestly, for some people, it should be.

Some of us need that kick in the butt to finally make a change. Others will become hyper-focused and start overresearching, avoiding every possible toxin and living by the book.

But I believe the 80/20 rule is where real, sustainable health lives. Be intentional and consistent 80% of the time, and leave room for joy, indulgence, and spontaneity the other 20%. Go on that vacation. Eat the cake. Then come home and get back into your groove.

This book isn't about fear; it is about empowerment. I want to teach you what's happening in your body and give you real-life tools you can use to support it. But I also want to remind you that only living within strict rules can create its own stress, and stress is one of the biggest disruptors to your health and your genes.

So breathe. Soften. Trust the process. Start small. Just make one to two changes every week, or two, or three, depending on how big and overwhelming the change is for you. Over time, those small shifts will snowball into a massive transformation.

The more consistent you are, the more permanent your genetic and cellular changes will become. And then … you'll be doing it. You'll be moving the needle from disease to wellness, no matter where you're starting from or how old you are.

I'm cheering you on every step of the way. If you're feeling ready to dive deeper into your health and truly support your body, I would be honored to walk that path with you or refer you to someone who could help in your area.

Through functional medicine testing, including hormone panels, gut microbiome testing, food sensitivity analysis, organic acids testing, methylation and genetic reports, or nutrient deficiencies, we can uncover what's really going on beneath the surface and create a plan that's uniquely tailored to you.

We can connect virtually through telemedicine, no matter where you are. If you're craving something more immersive and heart-centered, join us at one of our transformative retreats. These experiences are all about healing, connection, laughter, and truly reconnecting with yourself.

Think deep rest, nourishing food, beautiful surroundings, and a like-minded community. You deserve to feel vibrant, supported, and alive—so let's make it happen, together. DM me or contact our office.

Lastly, let me know what you love, what's challenging, and what's changing, what you don't like, and anything else that comes up for you. You've got this!

Your Journey Doesn't End Here, It's Just Getting Started

If this book resonated with you, then trust that something in you is already shifting. It could be a renewed sense of hope, a deeper connection to your body, or the realization that you're not alone in this.

Whatever it is, I want to remind you that this is only the beginning. Healing isn't a destination; it's a path. And while you now have the tools and insight to continue on that path, you don't have to walk it alone.

I created this book to be more than just information; I wanted it to feel like a conversation, a guide, and a gentle nudge back to your own innate wisdom.

Now that you've turned the last page, I want to invite you into a space where that connection continues. Where the ideas in these chapters become real-life practices, and where support, community, and transformation are always available to you.

If you're ready to take your healing to the next level, I would love to invite you to explore the resources, membership programs, and experiences I've created for exactly that purpose.

Whether you're craving deeper education, personalized guidance, or just a place to feel seen and supported, there's something here for you.

Let's Keep Going Together

For those seeking ongoing support, my monthly wellness membership program is a beautiful next step. Inside, you'll get access to deeper teachings, daily guides, weekly, monthly, six-month, and annual reassessments, protocols, monthly video trainings, and tools to help you integrate everything you've learned in this book at a pace that feels right for you.

It's also where we dive into new topics every month, ranging from detox to hormones to mindset to mitochondrial health. Most importantly, it's where you'll find a community of people walking the same path, cheering each other on, and doing the work together.

If you're seeking more personalized support, I also offer one-on-one coaching and functional medicine consulting. Whether you want to review labs, understand your symptoms on a deeper level, or create a custom healing plan that actually works for your body, I'm here to help. I work with clients all over the world, and every plan is tailored to your unique story, your biology, and your goals.

For those of you who feel called to go all in, pause, reset, and truly transform, I invite you to join me at one of my luxury wellness retreats. These retreats are not just about rest (though you'll get that too). They're about deep restoration, nervous system repair, and returning to a place of clarity, vitality, and alignment.

We blend education, movement, nature, healing modalities, food, and community to create something truly unforgettable. Plus, you'll get to explore a new country, go to some fun temples, meet enlightened shamans, and hopefully have a few awakening experiences of your own!

These are immersive, soul-nourishing experiences designed to help you reconnect with yourself and come home to your body in a way you may never have before.

You're Not Meant to Do This Alone

Healing doesn't happen in isolation. It happens in a community. It happens when you feel safe enough to be seen, supported enough to stay consistent, and inspired enough to keep going.

That's what I want to offer you—not just more content, but a relationship. A space to keep growing, asking questions, integrating new habits, and discovering what works for you.

If this book helped you, if it opened your eyes or shifted something in your heart, share it, talk about it, or gift it to someone you love. Your voice has power, and you never know who needs to hear exactly what you've just learned.

Research has shown something remarkable: the people we spend time with can greatly influence our own health. In one large study, having a close friend who is obese was linked to a

57% higher chance of becoming obese yourself. With siblings, the risk increased by 40%, and with a spouse, by 37%.[11]

This isn't about blame, shame, or judgment; it's about the powerful ripple effect our choices have on those around us. The way we live, eat, move, and care for ourselves can inspire others more than we realize.

You have the opportunity to be the spark, be the change, be the motivational force in your group or community that changes people's lives forever!

By making choices that support your well-being, you can quietly open the door for others to embark on their own transformation. One healthy choice can inspire another, and before you know it, it can cause entire circles of friends, families, and communities to shift toward greater well-being.

Health is best achieved together. Be the light in your community, the encouragement your loved ones need, and the proof that change is possible. The choices you make today might just be the turning point for someone you care about tomorrow.

---

[11] ByStaff Writer, By, and Staff Writer, "Friends, Family Can Influence Your Weight-for Good or Bad," Harvard T.H. Chan School of Public Health, November 22, 2024, https://hsph.harvard.edu/news/friends-and-family-can-influence-your-weight/#:~:text=Research%20has%20shown%20that%20a%20person's%20chance,is%20obese%2C%20according%20to%20the%20Thinfluence%20authors.

> To join the membership program, visit www.awakennowhealth.com/membership.
>
> To download free resources to keep you moving ahead, visit www.awakennowhealth.com/free-resources.
>
> You can also follow me on Instagram @awakennow or sign up for the weekly newsletter at www.awakennowhealth.com. Scroll to the bottom of the page, where I share wellness tips, real talk, and behind-the-scenes updates you won't find anywhere else.
>
> To book a one-on-one consultation with me, please visit www.awakennowhealth.com/contact-us.
>
> To learn more about the transformative retreats, visit www.awakennowhealth.com/retreats.

I believe in your ability to heal. I believe in your body's wisdom. And I believe that even the smallest steps, when taken with intention, can lead to massive transformation.

So stay curious, stay connected, and keep tuning into that voice inside you that's ready to feel better. I call my business AWAKEN NOW for a reason, because I want you to Awaken to your health, your life, and the world around you. I want you to AWAKEN TO YOU!

You're here for a reason, and your next chapter is already unfolding.

Let's begin.

With love and so much respect,

Marina Dabcevic Lac, DAOM, IFMCP

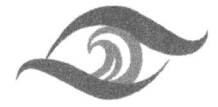

Acknowledgments

Writing this book has been an experience I will not soon forget. It's not just a collection of words, research, and stories; it's the sum of countless courses, conversations, lessons, challenges, and encouragements I've received along the way.

I have dreamed of writing a book for a long time now, but I never even allowed myself to say it out loud, so I did not share the fact that I was writing a book until I had spoken with Shanda at Transcendent Publishing to see if it was worth pursuing.

Learning and practicing what I preach has been a journey all its own. It's one thing to tell someone to jump, trust, and not be scared, and another to actually do it themselves. I can only forward my message, mission, and work into the world because of the extraordinary people who have been a part of my journey.

To my family—Mom, Dad, and my brother—you are my foundation. You challenge me in so many ways. You *always* tell me the honest truth, no matter how hard it is to hear. You love me no matter what, and you listen to me whenever I call. Thank you for always pushing me to do my best, even when I don't want to be pushed!

To my incredible kids, who are my mirrors and reflect to me all that is good and all that I still need to work on. I am learning, practicing, and evolving for you, through you, and with you. You are my everything, and I could not imagine my life without you. You chose me to be your mama, and I am beyond grateful for every day I have with you.

To Mike—you challenge me in ways that push me to grow, and I know that's one of the reasons I chose you for this journey. Thank you for holding down the fort with the kids while I edited, re-edited, and re-re-edited this manuscript. You stepped in, made me delicious meals, and made space for me to focus when it mattered most.

To my friend Elishah, who sat next to me one day by the pool and said, "Hey, you should write a functional medicine guide book," and four weeks later, the book was born! I am not sure what happened on that day, but the stars were aligned enough for me to overcome my self-doubt and start putting my fingers to a keyboard. Thank you!

To my predecessors—people I look up to and admire so much—Dr. Mark Hyman, Dr. Stacy Sims, Dr. Terry Wahls, Dr. Kara Fitzgerald, Dr. Gabrielle Lyon, Dr. Mindy Pelz, Dr. Ben Lynch, and so many more. Your work has inspired, challenged, and sharpened my thinking in ways that ripple throughout every chapter. Thank you for setting the bar high and for generously sharing your wisdom with the world.

To my friends who always listen to me, keep me on my toes, make me check in with myself when I need to be kind to myself, hug me when I cry, and make me laugh constantly. I don't know how I could do life without "Mother's Night Out," multiple family vacations, or weekend beach dates. You are my tribe, and thank you for never judging me when I …, well, let's say, fail at being a parent or mess up at being human!

Thank you, thank you, thank you!

To my patients and clients—you are my daily reminder of why this matters. Every breakthrough you've had, every setback you've faced with courage, and every story you've trusted me with has shaped how I see health, healing, and possibility. You are my teachers as much as I am yours.

To my colleagues, whom I call and rely on when cases get tough or I'm unsure of my way through a murky health picture. Thank you for helping me bounce ideas off of you and giving me clues on where to look next.

To Transcendent Publishing, Shanda, and Mary—thank you for believing in this project, guiding me through the process, and helping me bring it to life in a way that honors the vision I held from the very beginning. Your faith and dedication mean more than words can express. Mary, I will never forget the moment I saw the copyright page; it sent chills down my body as my fantasy became reality. Thank you, thank you, thank you both so incredibly much.

And to you, the reader—thank you for choosing to spend your time here. My hope is that you'll walk away not only with knowledge, but with a renewed belief in your ability to create the health, energy, and life you deserve.

This book is, in truth, a community effort. Every name here represents a thread in the fabric of these pages, and I am deeply, endlessly grateful for each one.

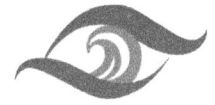

About the Author

Dr. Marina Dabcevic is a Board-certified Functional Medicine practitioner, licensed acupuncturist, and herbalist with over 25 years of experience in integrative health.

Born in Croatia and raised in Sydney, Australia, she began her healing journey early, driven by her own health challenges and a relentless curiosity about the body's deeper wisdom.

Dr. Marina holds a Master's Degree in Traditional Chinese Medicine and Acupuncture from Yo San University in Los Angeles, as well as a Doctorate in Acupuncture and Oriental Medicine from Bastyr University in Seattle, with a focus on oncology and chronic pain management.

Her training includes internships at top hospitals in China and a one-year clinical rotation at Skagit Valley Regional Cancer Care Center. She also holds a Bachelor's Degree in Homeopathy and a Diploma in Reflexology from Nature Care College in Australia.

But her passion didn't stop there. Frustrated by the limitations of conventional approaches, Dr. Marina pursued advanced studies in Functional Medicine through the Institute for Functional Medicine, Frequency-Specific Microcurrent therapy, and

Peptide Therapy. Her work is deeply rooted in connecting the physical, emotional, and spiritual aspects of health, empowering patients to understand the "why" behind their symptoms and reclaim their vitality.

Today, she runs her California-based practice, Awaken Now, where she helps clients from around the world address the root causes of their health concerns using personalized, science-backed protocols. When she's not working with patients or leading retreats, she's likely studying something new because her love for learning never stops.

To connect with Dr. Marina, explore her retreats, or join her wellness community, visit www.awakennowhealth.com or follow her on Instagram @awakennow.

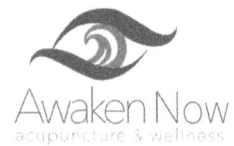

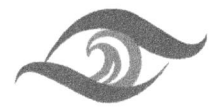

References

1. Bland, J. (2014). *The Disease Delusion: Conquering the Causes of Chronic Illness for a Healthier, Longer, and Happier Life.* Harper Wave.
2. Sims, S. (2016). *ROAR: How to Match Your Food and Fitness to Your Unique Female Physiology for Optimum Performance, Great Health, and a Strong, Lean Body for Life.* Rodale.
3. Sims, S. (2022). *Next Level: Your Guide to Kicking Ass, Feeling Great, and Crushing Goals Through Menopause and Beyond.* Rodale.
4. Kara, C. (2022). *Younger You: Reduce Your Bio Age and Live Longer, Better.* Ballantine Books.
5. Hyman, M. (2010). *Forever Young: The Science of Nutrigenomics for Glowing, Wrinkle-Free Skin and Radiant Health at Every Age.* Little, Brown Spark.
6. O'Bryan, T. (2016). *The Autoimmune Fix: How to Stop the Hidden Autoimmune Damage That Keeps You Sick, Fat, and Tired Before It Turns Into Disease.* Rodale.
7. Walker, M. (2017). *Why We Sleep: Unlocking the Power of Sleep and Dreams.* Scribner.

8. Lynch, B. (2018). *Dirty Genes: A Breakthrough Program to Treat the Root Cause of Illness and Optimize Your Health.* HarperOne.
9. Venn-Watson, S. (2021). *The Longevity Solution: Rediscovering Centuries-Old Secrets to a Healthy, Long Life.* [Often confused with "The Longevity Nutrient," referring to C15:0.]
10. Mayer, E. (2016). *The Mind-Gut Connection: How the Hidden Conversation Within Our Bodies Impacts Our Mood, Our Choices, and Our Overall Health.* Harper Wave.
11. Wahls, T. (2014). *The Wahls Protocol: A Radical New Way to Treat All Chronic Autoimmune Conditions Using Paleo Principles.* Avery.
12. Lipton, B. (2005). *The Biology of Belief: Unleashing the Power of Consciousness, Matter & Miracles.* Hay House.
13. Clear, J. (2018). *Atomic Habits: An Easy & Proven Way to Build Good Habits & Break Bad Ones.* Avery.
14. Fogg, B. J. (2019). *Tiny Habits: The Small Changes That Change Everything.* Houghton Mifflin Harcourt.
15. Attia, P. (2023). *Outlive: The Science and Art of Longevity.* Harmony.
16. Sinclair, D. (2019). *Lifespan: Why We Age—and Why We Don't Have To.* Atria Books.
17. Means, C. (2024). *Good Energy: The Surprising Connection Between Metabolism and Limitless Health.* Penguin Life.
18. Inchauspé, J. (2022). *Glucose Revolution: The Life-Changing Power of Balancing Your Blood Sugar.* Simon & Schuster.

19. Pelz, M. (2023). *Fast Like a Girl: A Woman's Guide to Using the Healing Power of Fasting to Burn Fat, Boost Energy, and Balance Hormones.* Hay House.

20. Minich, D. (2018). *The Rainbow Diet: A Holistic Approach to Radiant Health Through Foods and Supplements.* Conari Press.

21. Perlmutter, D. (2013). *Grain Brain: The Surprising Truth About Wheat, Carbs, and Sugar—Your Brain's Silent Killers.* Little, Brown Spark.

22. Hyman, M. (2016). *Eat Fat, Get Thin: Why the Fat We Eat Is the Key to Sustained Weight Loss and Vibrant Health.* Little, Brown Spark.

23. Cohen, A. (2020). *Non-Toxic: Guide to Living Healthy in a Chemical World.* Oxford University Press.

24. Pert, C. (1997). *Molecules of Emotion: The Science Behind Mind-Body Medicine.* Scribner.

25. Brach, E. (2018). *Stress Less, Accomplish More: Meditation for Extraordinary Performance.* Harmony.

26. Sovijärvi, O., Arina, T., & Halmetoja, J. (2018). *Biohacker's Handbook: Upgrade Yourself and Unleash Your Inner Potential.* Biohacker Center (BHC Inc.).

www.ingramcontent.com/pod-product-compliance
Lightning Source LLC
Chambersburg PA
CBHW070618030426
42337CB00020B/3843